Treatment of Substance Abuse
Psychosocial Occupational Therapy Approaches

Treatment of Substance Abuse
Psychosocial Occupational Therapy Approaches

Diane Gibson, MS, OTR
Editor

The Haworth Press
New York • London

Treatment of Substance Abuse: Psychosocial Occupational Therapy Approaches has also been published as *Occupational Therapy in Mental Health*, Volume 8, Number 2, 1988.

The Haworth Press, Inc. 10 Alice Street, Binghamton, NY 13904-1580
EUROSPAN/Haworth, 3 Henrietta Street, London WC2E 8LU England

LIBRARY OF CONGRESS
Library of Congress Cataloging-in-Publication Data

Treatment of substance abuse : psychosocial occupational therapy approaches / Diane Gibson, editor.

    p. cm.

    This title has also been published as: Occupational therapy in mental health, v. 8, no. 2, 1988.

    Bibliography: p.

    ISBN 0-86656-838-7

    1. Substance abuse – Treatment. 2. Occupational therapy. I. Gibson, Diane.

RC564.T74 1988

616.86′065152 – dc 19

88-21309
CIP

Treatment of Substance Abuse
Psychosocial Occupational Therapy Approaches

CONTENTS

ABOUT THE EDITOR

Diane Gibson, MS, OTR, is Director of Activity Therapy at The Sheppard and Enoch Pratt Hospital in Baltimore, Maryland, where her responsibilities include directing activity therapy treatment programs for approximately 350 hospitalized psychiatric patients of varying ages and diagnoses. She is also a senior faculty member at the Education Center, The Sheppard and Enoch Pratt Hospital. In addition to being the author of numerous publications in the occupational therapy field and a frequent lecturer on stress and management issues, she is the editor of *Occupational Therapy in Mental Health*.

Foreword

Treatment of Substance Abuse: Psychosocial Occupational Therapy Approaches provides an overview of contemporary assessment and rehabilitation of alcohol and chemical dependent substance abusers. Few articles in occupational therapy literature address this topic although many occupational therapists and other activity therapy staff work in substance abuse programs.

This special issue examines current polemics regarding the use of methadone versus abstinence oriented programs. The various articles provide insight into the role occupational therapy may play including behavioral and educational frames of reference as well as specific treatment modalities such as stress management, activities of daily living and leisure counseling.

Diane Gibson, MS, OTR
Editor

The Implementation
of an Occupational Therapy Program
in an Alcohol and Drug Dependency
Treatment Center

Melinda K. Stensrud, MS, OTR
Rosalie S. Lushbough, MS, OTR

SUMMARY. This project was designed to help establish occupational therapy as an appropriate and viable part of an adult alcohol and drug dependency rehabilitation program. Secondarily, its purpose was to meet the need for increased validation of the use of arts and crafts as effective and useful activities in occupational therapy sessions within this setting. Arts and crafts activity sessions were conducted twice a week with inpatients of an adult alcohol and drug dependency treatment center, and standard occupational therapy tools were used to measure the effect of this program on the rehabilitation of participating patients. Results showed that patients significantly improved over time in the areas of general, interpersonal, and task behaviors. CareUnit patient and staff feedback strongly supported the integration of occupational therapy into the overall treatment program. Implications of the appropriateness of occupational

Melinda K. Stensrud is a senior therapist, CareUnit (chemical dependency treatment center) of Western Medical Center, Anaheim, CA, and is pursuing a PhD at Walden University, Minneapolis, MN.

Rosalie S. Lushbough is a staff therapist at the Veterans Administration Hospital, Palo Alto, CA.

The authors would like to thank Dr. Lela Llorens, their major research advisor at San Jose State University, as well as the entire staff of San Jose Hospital's CareUnit for the opportunity to conduct this study.

Portions of this manuscript were included in the authors' thesis, submitted and accepted in partial fulfillment of the requirements of an MS degree from San Jose State University, San Jose, CA.

therapy in alcohol and drug dependency treatment centers are discussed.

Occupational therapy is as yet not a very well-known nor an established program component of drug and alcohol dependency treatment centers. A review of the literature revealed a paucity of information on occupational therapy programs in these settings. The most recent article that described such a program stated that the program's successes lay mainly in the areas of helping patients learn to handle frustration, increase awareness of personal strengths and weaknesses, share personal experiences and feelings, sort out priorities, ask for help, and learn new behavior patterns that would help them stay sober (Lindsay, 1983). To add to research regarding the effectiveness of occupational therapy in such a rehabilitation setting, the researchers evaluated a six week treatment program (given to a total of 41 patients) for one hour sessions two times a week at San Jose Hospital's CareUnit. The CareUnit is a 28 day inpatient program providing a broad range of treatment services including medical, psychological, educational, and counseling components for adults in treatment for drug and alcohol addiction. Projected benefits of this occupational therapy program for the participating patients were improved self-esteem, social relationships (including group cooperation), leisure time planning skills, problem solving, fine motor coordination, decision making, concentration, frustration tolerance, and an added measure of stimulating activity during their stay in the CareUnit.

The researchers have used the occupational behavior frame of reference as a guide to their practice and treatment intervention in this setting. "The occupational behavior frame of reference concerns the balance of play, work, and rest cycles as crucial to prevention and reduction of incapacities resulting from illness, trauma or occupation dysfunction. It is based on biological, sociological, psychological and occupational theory" (Llorens, 1984). Through the continuum of work (which includes paid and unpaid jobs and chores) and play (which includes social and leisure activities), a person learns the occupational roles needed to become competent in society. The researchers believe that this theoretical framework may be particularly appropriate for this patient population in that it addresses the problems of performance of life roles; the functional skill components (i.e., motor, sensory, cognitive, social, and psychological) required to perform life roles; and the maintenance of an optimal balance in the occupational areas of self-care, play, work, leisure, and learning.

The researchers' treatment program consisted of the use of arts and crafts as purposeful activities. The decision to use these activities was made in response to the request of the CareUnit's Program Manager and primary alcoholism therapist, who perceived the CareUnit's current program as using primarily verbal and written treatment modalities and thus lacking task-oriented creative activities. Commonly used evaluation tools (see Aim of the Program) revealed changes in the subjects' general, interpersonal and/or task behaviors while engaged in occupational therapy arts and crafts activities, as well as their feelings about their performance during these activities. The researchers' aim was to demonstrate that this treatment program was an effective and viable part of the overall CareUnit program.

This paper describes a six week occupational therapy program that was designed to treat inpatients at San Jose Hospital's Care-Unit, a chemical dependency treatment program. The occupational therapy intervention was limited to arts and crafts for purposes of the study in an effort to isolate the effects of these modalities. The paper addresses the effectiveness of arts and crafts activities in this setting and reports the behavioral and subjective responses of patients to the occupational therapy intervention. A description of the program is presented, followed by a discussion of the outcome and implications for future occupational therapy programs and research.

DESCRIPTION OF THE PROGRAM

Subjects

All 41 participants in this study were inpatients at San Jose Hospital's CareUnit. A typical patient profile revealed a gamut of possible personal characteristics with no exclusion criteria on the basis of sex, race, religion, education, financial status, or cultural heritage. All participants, however, were adults (18 years of age or over) who had alcohol and/or drug abuse problems and the means to pay for the CareUnit program through their own funds, through an employee assistance program, or through a third party payer, such as private health insurance or Medicare.

All patients in the CareUnit were invited to participate in the occupational therapy sessions. Selection of the subjects was determined by their own decision to participate in this study after attending an inservice program given by the researchers on the philosophy, value, and treatment modalities of occupational therapy. Those patients admitted to the CareUnit after the initial inservice program were given a briefing on the meaning and relevance of occupational therapy to their treatment program as well as printed material that described occupational therapy in greater detail. Agreement to participate in the study was confirmed by the patient's signing a consent form which described the occupational therapy program, the research design and procedure, and each subject's rights and obligations as a participant in the study. CareUnit staff members encouraged patient participation in the occupational therapy program as an equally valid and relevant part of their overall treatment. The researchers set, as a minimum treatment program, at least 3 sessions (two weeks) and a maximum program of 8 sessions (four weeks) for a subject's results to be used for statistical analysis. Exclusion criteria included destructive or overly disruptive behavior to self or others, and/or recommendation by a CareUnit staff member that a patient not participate in occupational therapy.

A Typical Occupational Therapy Session

Occupational therapy sessions were held for one hour twice a week in the afternoons and were open to patients who wished to participate. Both researchers led each session, which generally had between eight and fifteen participants. A variety of structured and unstructured tasks were used as treatment modalities. Structured tasks were distinguished from unstructured tasks in terms of having a specific outcome, detailed procedures necessary to accomplish the task, and certain types of materials used (Clark & Cross, 1982). For example, wooden coat racks were made from kits which supplied simple step-by-step directions and only the materials necessary to complete the project. In contrast, the activity wherein participants were instructed to create clay animals representing themselves is an example of an unstructured task. Participants had to decide what they were going to make and how they were going to make it, as the material was pliable and suggested no particular outcome.

At the beginning of each session, the occupational therapists reiterated the purposes of occupational therapy, which included enhancing patients': (1) *self-understanding*, i.e., handling frustration, identifying and expressing feelings appropriately, acknowledging progress and bolstering self-confidence, becoming more independent, and following through on tasks toward accomplishment of their goals; (2) *interpersonal and communication skills*, i.e., controlling impulses, initiating appropriate contacts within a group and one-to-one, listening more and acknowledging the feelings of others, being assertive, asking for help and support, and accepting feedback from others; (3) *work performance skills*, i.e., organizing one's workspace and pacing oneself, listening to and following directions better, trying new things, making decisions for oneself, using projects to channel feelings (such as anger), and learning to break large goals into small, manageable steps; and (4) *leisure time skills*, such as increasing awareness of one's leisure interests and managing one's leisure time better by developing new hobbies and leisure interests.

After a review of the purposes, the therapists described the activity and the steps involved, gave time limits, and approximately ten minutes prior to the close of each hour the group was invited to audit their individual and group processes.

The therapists tried to create a relaxed and unthreatening atmosphere where people felt at ease and accepted, although inappropriate behavior was discouraged by way of open feedback offered by patients and therapists alike.

AIM OF PROGRAM
AND HOW IT WAS CARRIED OUT

These series of occupational therapy sessions were designed to study the effectiveness of occupational therapy as an integral part of the CareUnit program. This evaluative study examined how well the occupational therapy program met its objectives. The researchers' criteria for an effective program included the following guidelines:

1. Patient improvement would be observable and documented (using the various evaluation tools) specifically in general, interpersonal and task behaviors as they reflect a balanced and sober lifestyle.
2. Patients would respond positively to the occupational therapy program as shown by their responses on the occupational therapy questionnaire.
3. The CareUnit staff would deem occupational therapy evaluation and treatment as a valuable and integral part of the overall program.
4. The CareUnit staff would request continuation of occupational therapy services after the formal program evaluational study was completed.

Each of these criteria was met, as outlined in the Outcomes section.

The following data collection tools were used to gather this information: the *Comprehensive Occupational Therapy Evaluation* (*COTE Scale*, Brayman & Kirby, 1982), the *Activity Laboratory Questionnaire* (Fidler, 1982), Cynkin's (1979) *Activities Clock*, the researchers' *Occupational Therapy Questionnaire*, and the *Initial Evaluation Interview* (Ehrenberg, 1982). This combination of evaluation tools was selected because it allowed for objective assessment as well as patients' self-report. Chemically dependent and alcohol patients typically displayed impaired social and interpersonal skills, low self-esteem, poor time management and difficulty getting places on time, problems in carrying out job duties, unclear values and unreasonable goals, and unbalanced lifestyles of work, self-care, rest and leisure activities. The *COTE* scale objectively assessed performance in these areas; Fidler's *Activity Laboratory Questionnaire* assessed patients' subjective views about their task performance; Cynkin's *Activities Clock* guided the patients toward developing a balance in the work, self-care, rest and leisure activities of daily life; the *Occupational Therapy Questionnaire* helped the patients proactively consider how they would like their treatment program to be in the future; and Ehrenberg's *Initial Evaluation Interview* helped patients integrate past work and education experience with future goals.

The most comprehensive data gathering instrument was the *COTE Scale*, which was completed by the researchers after each treatment session. This scale measured changes in general, interpersonal, and task behaviors over time.

The researchers also completed the *Initial Evaluation Interview* from Ehrenberg's *Comprehensive Assessment Process*. Initial interviews were arranged soon after each patient entered the CareUnit, with both researchers and one patient at a time in attendance. These interviews were conducted in order to establish rapport between the researchers and each patient, and to give the patient an opportunity to share information about him or herself regarding family life, education, work history, recreational interests, and anything else the patient wanted to share. The information obtained from these interviews was analyzed for demographic details of the population being studied.

During both the initial interview and a discharge planning session, patients were asked to complete an *Activities Clock* reflecting a typical weekday schedule to illustrate how they organized their days' time prior to admission and how they proposed to do so to help maintain sobriety post-discharge from the CareUnit. After the patients had completed their post-discharge time use plan, reinforcing information was given by the researchers on the value of maintaining a healthy balance between their daily work, sleep, self-care, social, and leisure activities. Comparisons of the pre- and proposed post-discharge time use plans were statistically analyzed to reveal any changes in each patient's orientation toward time management.

After each week of treatment, patients were asked to complete the *Activity Laboratory Questionnaire*. The purpose of monitoring subjects' responses over time was for both the researchers and the subjects to gain insight into how they felt about their performance while doing the activities, factors that might have influenced that performance, and the activities they enjoyed doing the least or the most. An analysis of variance and a post hoc trend analysis on an item by item basis was conducted to reveal trends which occurred within the group of subjects.

During each patient's discharge planning session, the researchers administered the *Occupational Therapy Questionnaire* which asked the following questions:

1. If you had been given the choice, would you have chosen to have occupational therapy as part of your CareUnit treatment program?
2. Would you have preferred more time in occupational therapy? If yes, how much more time?
3. Would you have preferred occupational therapy sessions to be scheduled at different times of the day? If yes, when?
4. If given a choice, what activities would you have preferred to take part in other than occupational therapy?

The responses were analyzed with a simple Chi square. The results of this questionnaire may be helpful in guiding researchers and CareUnit staff in planning future occupational therapy programs.

OUTCOMES

Apparent Value of the Program

Results of the *COTE* scale analysis revealed that there was improvement (i.e., better scores per person over time) in all three areas covered: general, interpersonal, and task behaviors. Total scores showed that the mean errors per person decreased by 4.44 from each patient's first to last session. (See Table 1.) These are the results that the researchers attempted to achieve by way of this treatment program, however, the improvements in behavior seen over time must be considered as resulting from the effectiveness of the overall CareUnit program and the improved physical health of the individual, as well as from the occupational therapy program.

Fidler's *Activity Laboratory Questionnaire* revealed the following information regarding how the patients felt about their performance; which parts of the activity process were most pleasant and

TABLE 1

SUMMARY OF OBJECTIVE FINDINGS

	BASELINE		RESULTS	IMPLICATIONS
COTE Scale	Scores: first session		last session	
	General behavior: 1.94		1.11	Lower scores imply significant improvement in general, interpersonal and task behaviors over 8 sessions.
	Interpersonal:	2.59	1.00	
	Task:	3.06	1.23	
	Total	7.59	3.34	
Activities Clock		Hours	Hours	
	Sleep	5.63	6.75	Patients learned to better plan their time use toward a more balanced lifestyle in terms of work, rest and leisure activities. Note: patients included aftercare 12-step meetings (e.g. A.A./N.A./C.A.) in their work hours.
	Work	7.88	9.00	
	Leisure	6.00	3.88	
	Chores	2.25	2.38	
	Social	2.24	2.00	

unpleasant; which activities they liked best; and what factors influenced their performance the most.

Most patients (63.4%) thought they did quite well on all the occupational therapy activities, and perceptions of their performance did not vary much over time. Given that the activities chosen were purposefully simple, it was not surprising that most patients were able to perform to their satisfaction on these various tasks. It was interesting to observe that patients who appeared to have low self-esteem still rated their performance as generally good.

It was revealed that the participants in this program, responding to the question regarding what they found to be the most pleasant part of the occupational therapy sessions, were most appreciative of opportunities to be physically active, and for the chance to get to know each other better. The patients found that the physical and sensory aspects of the arts and crafts activities were stimulating and provided variety from the rest of the CareUnit program.

There was an even distribution of participants who felt that the most unpleasant aspect of the occupational therapy sessions was either nothing at all or a lack of time, indicating relatively positive feelings toward occupational therapy. This, combined with the other write-in responses, has led the researchers to determine that, although the activities were neither excessively mentally nor physically challenging, they were appropriate given that their purpose was to provide successful short-term task activities which would enhance the personal meaningfulness of the didactic material in the CareUnit program.

The data revealed that there was no strong preference for one activity over another, nor can one deduce that nonstructured activities were significantly more or less popular than the structured activities. By way of observation rather than data analysis, the researchers have surmised that individuals tended to consistently prefer either the specificity of detailed directions given in structured activities or the lack of rigidity and defined procedures that characterized unstructured activities.

The response overwhelmingly favored by the patients to the question regarding what factors most influenced their performance was "the desire to do a good job." This choice took precedence even over external factors, such as being observed by others and distracting noise. This response seemed to be in line with the CareUnit staff's viewpoint that alcoholics often have perfectionist tendencies and are also frequently "workaholics." The researchers noticed how frustrating it was for patients who felt limited in their task completion either by lack of skill or time.

Fidler's *Activity Laboratory Questionnaire* was found to be very useful in monitoring the patients' internal reactions to their task processes. It was adaptable to the comparison of two or more activities and it helped the patients to identify their feelings. The analyzed data from both the *Activity Laboratory Questionnaire* and the *Occupational Therapy Questionnaire* clearly revealed that the patients enjoyed occupational therapy as an integral part of their CareUnit program. Two-thirds of the respondents noted that they would have preferred having from three to five hours of occupational therapy per week, instead of the two hour per week schedule. The researchers believe that the *Occupational Therapy Questionnaire* effectively gathers feedback on how well occupational therapy is meeting patient needs, and would recommend continued use of this questionnaire.

Cynkin's *Activities Clock* proved to be a useful tool in allowing patients to review both how they structured their daily time use while using drugs and/or alcohol, and how they planned to use their time while sober and drug-free. The data showed that in the area of sleep, the patients averaged only 5.63 hours per night prior to admission into the CareUnit. According to Coon (1983), only eight percent of the population averages five hours of sleep per night; most people sleep on a familiar seven to eight hour per night schedule. During discussions with the patients that involved their time use plans, the researchers suggested that they attempt to bring their lives into balance by scheduling sleep, work, leisure, social, and chore activities to their greatest physical, mental, spiritual, and emotional benefit. In planning their post-discharge schedules, most patients decided they would increase their sleep and work hours and that their time spend in leisure and social activities would be less. By adding to their work time, it is not necessarily correct to assume that they would be staying at their jobs longer, but that they would probably be attending regular Alcoholics Anonymous/Narcotics Anonymous/Cocaine Anonymous meetings and other activities related to their aftercare and sobriety (as these meetings were classified as "work" for the purposes of the study).

The researchers feel that Cynkin's *Activities Clock*, because it graphically displays the information, has been valuable to the patients, who have sometimes expressed surprise after examining their time use habits and have recognized the need to restructure their daily schedules thereafter.

Given that the objective of this study was to develop and implement an occupational therapy program of evaluation and treatment for adult alcohol and drug dependent patients, and to collect data regarding the effectiveness of this program, the CareUnit staff, the CareUnit patients, and the researchers all agree that the addition of the occupational therapy program was effective and valuable. The CareUnit Medical Director and the therapists cited patient treatment goals (from occupational therapy evaluations) and observations regarding patient behaviors (communicated during daily sessions and weekly staffings) as particularly helpful in assessing each patient's overall functioning, progress and treatment strategies. Due to the success of the occupational therapy intervention, the CareUnit/ Comprehensive Care Corporation staff formally requested continuation and expansion of this program.

IMPLICATIONS

Based on the results of this study, the authors support the integration of programs that utilize arts and crafts in addition to other modalities, because they provide short, successful, focussed, one hour sessions that result in a tangible product. Also, doing arts and crafts taps into the more creative processes of the brain, specifically in the right hemisphere, which allows both hemispheres to integrate information and experiences, thereby expanding learning capabilities. The authors support Kielhofner's (1983) opinion about crafts:

> Craft is one of the most powerful traditions in occupational therapy, but its use as a context of therapy has unfortunately declined. Hall, Haas, and Dunton were early occupational therapy proponents who advocated craft as one of the most uplifting and organizing human experiences, since it combined order, precision, creativity, planning and concrete reality. They perceived a need for occupational therapists to be thorough crafts-persons. The ideal of the occupational therapist as craftsperson seems to be dying, and this is a tremendous loss to the art of the field.

The occupational therapy clinic, in contrast to today's technologically oriented health care system based on the medical model, provides a unique and important contribution to patient care.

The authors believe that further research is needed with a larger sample of this population to attempt to replicate the effectiveness results of this study. They also believe that an expanded occupational therapy program would reinforce the didactic material by giving patients the opportunity to effectively use newly acquired concepts in skill-building classes. An ideal occupational therapy program might include a task performance group where personal goals are met; regular physical conditioning groups to support the process of detoxification and utilization of new stress management techniques; leisure planning and time management groups to help patients develop aftercare plans that reflect personal values and balanced, sober lifestyles; assertion training to foster critical skills for relationship building and to encourage honest, direct self-expression; and stress management workshops which employ progressive muscle relaxation techniques and help patients identify or practice newly acquired coping mechanisms. Regular recreational groups and outings would encourage patients to play and self-reward and would help them to connect with community resources. One-to-one time could also help individuals to clarify values as they relate to personal goals and career aspirations. Other topics might include money management, personal health and grooming, planning and preparing meals, making living arrangements, homemaking, public transportation, and seeking and keeping a job. The occupational therapist's unique service should continue to provide the patient with a holistic treatment program, aligned with the professionally prescribed goals of the multidisciplinary team and the patient, and free from overlap with other services.

LIMITATIONS

Limitations identified by the researchers include:

1. The possibility that since the researchers also implemented the occupational therapy program and gathered the data, they may have introduced personal biases into the study.
2. Changes from the participants' baseline behavior shown by the results of the *COTE* scale analysis may not be directly attributable to occupational therapy but may result from the combined therapies and experiences in the CareUnit. Baseline behavior was defined as that which participants exhibited during their first session in occupational therapy.
3. The possibility that since some participants in the study attended occupational therapy sessions irregularly, the consistency with which their behavior was observed and recorded was diminished. However, those who attended fewer than three sessions were not included in the data analysis.

4. The fact that, due to irregular participant attendance and a low CareUnit census, the researchers had a smaller sample size than hoped for, which could lessen the value of the results of the study.

5. The fact that the patient sample was nonrandom, and most participants came from a limited geographical area, thereby limiting the generalizability of the results.

SUMMARY

The researchers conducted this study in order to contribute to the occupational therapy profession's literature and data base regarding the effectiveness of arts and crafts activities with this particular population.

It was found that two one hour arts and crafts activity sessions per week provided the patients with a welcome change from the normal regimen of many lectures and verbal groups per day that were primarily analytical, confrontational, and sedentary. Results indicated that patients generally enjoyed their experiences in occupational therapy and felt good about their performance on most of the activities. Occupational therapy sessions appeared to provide these patients with a release of tension, a chance to be active, and a relaxing therapeutic milieu that helped them improve social skills (i.e., decreased isolation, enhanced self-esteem, and increased bonding with peers, staff and the CareUnit/A.A./N.A. programs). Results also showed that patients intended to structure their time differently (i.e., more balanced in terms of hours per day spent in work, sleep, chores, social, and leisure activities) after discharge from the CareUnit than prior to admission. This study revealed that general, interpersonal, and task behaviors of participating patients improved over time. All participants who responded to a questionnaire stated that they would have chosen to include occupational therapy in their treatment program, 67% requesting an increase in the hours per week of occupational therapy as well as requesting physical activities in the overall program.

The CareUnit staff invited the occupational therapists to continue this program in order to improve the quality of the patients' treatment and to facilitate and encourage the maintenance of a healthy and sober life.

The researchers highly promote the utilization of the results of this study to further develop occupational therapy's role in other alcohol and drug dependency treatment settings.

REFERENCES

Brayman, S.J., & Kirby, T. (1982). The comprehensive occupational therapy evaluation. In B.J. Hemphill (Ed.), *The evaluative process in psychiatric occupational therapy* (pp. 211-226, 381-388). Thorofare, NJ: Charles B. Slack, Inc.

Clark, E.N., & Cross, M.S. (1982). The creative clay test and an exploration of task structure. In B.J. Hemphill (Ed.), *The evaluative process in psychiatric occupational therapy* (pp. 211-226, 381-388). Thorofare, NJ: Charles B. Slack, Inc.

Coon, D. (1983). *Introduction to psychology: Exploration and application*. San Francisco: West Publishing Co.

Cynkin, S. (1979). *Toward health through activities*. Boston: Little, Brown and Company.

Ehrenberg, F. (1982). Comprehensive assessment process: A group evaluation. In B.J. Hemphill (Ed.), *The evaluative process in psychiatric occupational therapy* (pp. 155-168, 363-364). Thorofare, NJ: Charles B. Slack, Inc.

Fidler, G.S. (1982). The activity laboratory: A structure for observing and assessing perceptual, integrative, and behavioral strategies. In B.J. Hemphill (Ed.), *The evaluative process in psychiatric occupational therapy* (pp. 195-208, 379-380). Thorofare, NJ: Charles B. Slack, Inc.

Kielhofner, G. (1983). *Health through occupation: Theory and practice in occupational therapy* (p. 307). Philadelphia: F.A. Davis Company.

Lindsay, W.P. (1983). The role of the occupational therapist treatment of alcoholism. *American Journal of Occupational Therapy*, *37*, 36-43.

Llorens, L.A. (1984). Theoretical conceptualizations of occupational therapy: 1960-1982. *Occupational Therapy and Mental Health*, *4*(2), 1-14.

Occupational Therapy Intervention in the Treatment of Alcoholics

Catherine L. Cassidy

SUMMARY. The first section of this article will provide the rationale for all occupational therapists to learn extensively about the disease of alcoholism regardless of area of practice or type of agency where employed. It will offer suggestions on how this learning can take place. The second section will take an historic look at occupational therapy literature documenting the use of occupational therapy in alcoholism rehabilitation from 1941 to the present. It will describe modalities currently being used by occupational therapists in alcoholism rehabilitation and discuss expansion of occupational therapy in this practice area.

TREATMENT OF ALCOHOLICS IN THE GENERAL PATIENT POPULATION

Occupational therapists live and work in a society pervaded by alcohol and alcoholism. Statistics compiled in National Council on Alcoholism (NCA) publications based on government figures (NIAAA, 4th Report to Congress, 1981) are overwhelming. With at least 10,000,000 alcoholics in the U.S. (one in ten adult Americans), the NCA ranks alcoholism second only to cardiovascular diseases in number of victims but also ranks it second to last in finan-

---

Catherine L. Cassidy is affiliated with Mills-Peninsula Hospitals, Burlingame, CA.

The author gratefully acknowledges the editing efforts of Ann MacRae, an assistant professor of Occupational Therapy at San Jose State University, San Jose, California.

17

cial support given based on dollars/victim revenue spent (No Comment Fact Sheet, 1981). It is also estimated that each alcoholic negatively effects an average of four other persons (NCA, Alcohol and Alcoholism: Facts, Figures, and Findings, 1982) sufficiently for these other victims of alcoholism to require counseling and/or support to recover. Many of these effects are serious and become long-standing medical and emotional health problems for these individuals.

The direct or indirect effects of alcoholism can be found in every area of our society and, therefore, in every area of occupational therapy practice. Occupational therapists working in medical and psychiatric facilities treat alcoholic patients daily. A disproportionate number of alcoholics seek help in general medical and psychiatric facilities because they experience more problems than normal drinkers and because they try to avoid the stigma attached to receiving help from alcoholism agencies (Weschler & Rohman, 1982). The problem with this approach is that the symptom is treated, not the disease of alcoholism. The U.S. health care system is strongly impacted by alcoholism. At least 20% of all hospitalized persons have a significant alcohol problem regardless of presenting problem of admitting diagnosis with $12.8 billion spent annually to treat alcohol related health problems (Kinney & Leaton, 1983). The majority of these patients, nine out of ten, who come into contact with the U.S. health care system go without the primary problem, alcoholism, being diagnosed or treated (Whitfield & Williams, cited in Smith, 1983). With continued drinking the diagnosed symptom and potentially others will exacerbate and be treated again. This cycle will continue until the underlying alcoholism is diagnosed and treated. Occupational therapists, both psychiatric and medical, and other health care professionals working in hospital systems are in a position to correct this situation by understanding the disease of alcoholism more fully.

Occupational therapists who work in special areas of interest need also be aware of the effects of alcoholism on their clients. Becoming addicted to alcohol profoundly compounds the already significant problems presented by these clients. This includes occupational therapists working with pediatric, adolescent, female, and geriatric populations. Pediatric and female clients are impacted by the fact that fetal alcohol syndrome (FAS) is the third leading cause of mental retardation and is preventable. FAS children also suffer from physical abnormalities, developmental delays, and hyperactivity (NIAAA, 4th Report, 1981). Beyond the real dangers of FAS, 34% of female alcoholics are at risk to also be addicted to prescription drugs. An estimated 35% to 50% of alcoholics are female (NIAAA, 4th Report, 1981). Adolescents who drink, and 80% of them do, are particularly vulnerable to develop alcoholism, showing addiction with smaller amounts and a more rapid progression of the disease. By age 13, 54.5% of adult problem drinkers had their first drink (NCA, Alcohol and Teenagers Fact Sheet, 1983). Two types of alcoholics are found among geriatric patients. Some have had a long history of alcoholism and have survived to old age. There are also a growing number who turn to alcohol to cope with the multiple problems of aging and develop late onset alcoholism (Buys & Saltman, 1982). Alcohol problems in the elderly are further complicated by the potential for drug interactions between the alcohol and over-the-counter and/or prescription medications (Dobie, 1978).

Occupational therapists have a role to play in providing information for correct diagnosis and treatment of alcoholics. The first area is in documenting observations of or reports of patient drinking or preoccupation with drinking. While a patient is engaged in an occupational therapy task, he or she may become engrossed enough in the task to verbally or behaviorally divulge signs of a possible drinking problem. For example, a patient may be in the hospital and offering drinks to visitors and peers and grandiosely share this information during occupational therapy. He or she may also make verbal references to having a high tolerance for alcohol, having had blackouts, or other signs of alcoholism. The length of occupational therapy treatment ranging from fifteen to sixty minutes gives occupational therapists more patient contact time in which to make these observations than other hospital personnel. Documenting these observations will give other health care professionals all the pertinent information for evaluation and treatment purposes.

Health care facilities not designed to deal with alcoholism are not prepared to give the specialized treatment required by alcoholics. Occupational therapists and other professionals working in such agencies can serve these patients by learning about alcoholism treatment facilities in their community so appropriate treatment referrals can be made (Dorsch & Talley, 1973; Chappel & Schnoll, 1977; Weschler & Rohman, 1982).

Education of health care professionals regarding the disease of alcoholism is a forerunner to their being able to identify and treat alcoholics (DiCicco & Unterberger, 1977; Bailey, 1970; Dorsch & Talley, 1973). Increasing the time spent on alcoholism in occupational therapy basic education programs wherever possible is one way to address this issue. Current time spent ranges from zero to six hours in entry level programs (Cassidy, 1985). Increasing the offerings at the continuing education level for occupational therapists on alcoholism would benefit those wanting increased knowledge and those already in practice. Occupational therapists can also learn about the disease and current treatment strategies by attending workshops presented by alcoholism specialists.

A final element in enabling occupational therapists to work effectively with alcoholics is to allow them to review their attitudes toward alcoholics and be sure they hold those which are optimistic and empathetic for recovery. Education alone does not ensure positive attitudes toward alcoholic patients (Chappel & Schnoll, 1977; Weschler & Rohman, 1982). Increasing the number of internships in alcoholism treatment centers would add substance to educational efforts regarding alcoholism and would allow occupational therapists opportunity to review their attitudes toward alcoholics in a clinical setting. This is an excellent means of dealing with emotional issues around alcoholism especially when combined with seminars during the internship to discuss issues and emotions which surface while treating alcoholic patients (Fisher et al., 1975). Occupational therapists would benefit from attending a variety of Alcoholics Anonymous and Al-Anon meetings to learn more about this disease and the recovery process at the "grass roots" level.

It is sincerely hoped that other health care professionals will join occupational therapists in this effort.

TREATMENT OF ALCOHOLICS IN ALCOHOLISM REHABILITATION

Although direct intervention by occupational therapists in alcoholism rehabilitation is documented in the literature, a 30 year literature review shows this information to be limited. Early occupational therapist intervention relied heavily on the therapeutic use of crafts in long-term programs working with "skid-row" alcoholics (Marston, 1942). Short-term facilities emphasized the value of a balance between work and leisure to patients but did not find crafts successful (Hossack, 1952). By 1953 Doniger reports occupational therapists teaching relaxation techniques to alcoholics and becoming involved in patient aftercare. Welsh (1959) reports therapists using psychiatric occupational therapy methods to select the most therapeutically beneficial activity for each patient. Occupational therapists' reports of observations of patients engaged in activities had diagnostic value. Prevocational exploration and a variety of groups were used as treatment methods by occupational therapists. Therapists also began to increase effectiveness of treatment by gaining an increased understanding of the disease process and the psychodynamics of alcoholism. In 1971, Zimberg, Lipscomb, and Davis reported the use of occupational therapy in the treatment of alcoholics in an urban ghetto setting.

Current use of occupational therapy in this area of treatment practice is minimal. The American Occupational Therapy Association's (A.O.T.A.'s) 1986 Member Data Survey shows 1.1% or 356 registered occupational therapists and 2.4% of certified occupational therapy assistants or 186 working nationwide in alcoholism rehabilitation.

Description of an occupational therapy program in an alcoholism treatment center is based on a review of occupational therapy and alcoholism treatment literature and this author's experience in an adolescent alcohol and drug abuse treatment center. Alcoholism treatment literature abounds with the use of behavioral techniques in the treatment of alcoholism. One article is representative of the literature (Agne & Paolucci, 1982). In "A Holistic Approach to an Alcoholic Treatment Program," the authors describe a program of nutrition counseling, regular exercise, stress reduction techniques, recreational pursuits, individual and family counseling, and regular attendance at AA meetings. Occupational therapists have the training and skills to offer intervention in several of these areas.

The occupational therapist is part of a treatment team in a milieu setting offering intervention in the evaluation, rehabilitation, and aftercare phases of treatment. Evaluation of alcoholics by occupational therapists is not standardized or consistent. In this phase is the beginning of contributions to overall staff evaluation of patients through observation of patients in activities and reporting these observations in team meetings. This process continues throughout treatment. Some occupational therapists (Maiorana, 1983) administer the Michigan Alcoholism Screening Test while others (Lindsay, 1983) use the self-image collage for evaluation. In using the self-image collage the occupational therapist can observe the patient in problem solving, eye-hand coordination, and direction following tasks as well as learn about the patient's sense of self. The patient is also given an initial opportunity to share his or her work with other members of the community and begin group communication skills.

In the rehabilitation phase of treatment occupational therapy provides several means for patients to identify and express emotions. Art is one such modality that can be used in individual or group projects (Smith & Glickstein, 1980-81). Other such modalities are projective writing exercises and poetry writing.

In addition to sharing patient attitudes and behaviors with other staff members, occupational therapists give continuous feedback to patients by reinforcing socially acceptable behavior and correcting nonreality oriented attitudes and perceptions (Blum & Blum, cited in Lindsay, 1983). Attitudes and behaviors learned in drinking and using times are well ingrained in alcoholics and persist into sobriety. Confronting the attitudes and behaviors which are inappropriate in sobriety and which contribute to relapse is an ongoing process throughout treatment. Occupational therapists are in a unique position to observe and confront these behaviors as they surface more often when patients are otherwise concentrating on tasks or in the less structured environments of outings. Successful completion of tasks in occupational therapy also helps patients develop a sense of competency (Macdonald, 1976) and increases self-esteem.

Of continuing value in all phases of treatment is the structure offered to patients (Maiorana & Lindsay, 1983; Larson, 1971) in occupational therapy groups and the opportunity to learn group cohesion and communication skills. Either by the therapeutic use of crafts or other group interventions alcoholics can improve planning, problem solving, fine eye-hand coordination, stress management, memory, time management, and leisure skills enhancing activities of daily living skills. Cooking groups can be used to teach cooking skills to lower functioning patients or to teach group participation skills with higher functioning patients. Prevocational and vocational evaluation of patients can also be done by occupational therapists (Larson, 1971; Lindsay, 1983). Experientially the value of vocational evaluation in early treatment was limited as other treatment issues focusing on establishing basic sobriety took precedence over work-related issues.

Final phase of treatment takes place after the patient has been discharged from the center. Barth (1980) describes occupational therapy in aftercare which takes place from one to three years after inpatient treatment. Therapists assist alcoholics in avoiding backsliding into old coping styles and drinking. Occupational therapy expertise helps clients take techniques on how to live without relying on alcohol and incorporate them into daily life. Further personal growth is facilitated by creative-expressive techniques to increase awareness of personal motivation and feelings. Shannon (1972) joins other occupational therapy writers in encouraging occupational therapists to do more of the community based, reality oriented occupational therapy by assisting human beings in the adaptive process which would include working with alcoholics.

Occupational therapy offers practical, common sense, activity oriented intervention with alcoholics giving them a means of learning skills needed in sobriety while still in some phase of treatment. Occupational therapy intervention also places strong emphasis on the value and potential of each individual in treatment (Lidz, 1966; Meyer, 1922 & 1937; Engelhardt, 1977).

During all phases of treatment alcoholics are oriented to membership in Alcoholics Anonymous (A.A.) which has the most successful approach to maintaining sobriety. A.A. is rich in common sense tactics and slogans that help alcoholics maintain sobriety over extensive periods of time. Fundamental in its appeal to alcoholics is the acceptance or feeling of value each alcoholic receives within the

A.A. fellowship regardless of life status or length of sobriety (Kurtz, 1979; Alcoholics Anonymous, 1952).

Sharing common sense approach to sobriety as well as holding high regard for the potential of each alcoholic gives occupational therapy and A.A. a kinship that is unique. Occupational therapy intervention with alcoholics who are in treatment is seen as valuable to patients who are being "groomed" as members of A.A. Occupational therapists provide structured activities and teach skills during treatment that can be continued once the alcoholic is out of treatment. The variety of these groups has been described in another part of this paper.

Increasing the use of occupational therapy in alcoholism rehabilitation will be a challenge. There is competition for health care dollars and professional rivalry due to misunderstanding of professional roles. Several areas need to be addressed in this process. The educational suggestions in the first section of this paper will give occupational therapists the knowledge and understanding of the disease needed to work with alcoholic patients. All occupational therapists need specific knowledge of dual diagnosis, i.e., patient with diagnosis of alcoholism and other significant medical or psychiatric diagnosis.

A national level program giving full description of occupational therapy interventions available for use with alcoholic patients would be useful to occupational therapists attempting to establish occupational therapy service in alcohol treatment centers. This intervention needs to be based on current treatment strategies used in alcoholism rehabilitation and occupational therapy theory.

Occupational therapists need to conduct research to show scientifically the value of occupational therapy intervention in alcoholism rehabilitation. Third party reimbursement sources also need to be shown the cost effectiveness of occupational therapy intervention with alcoholics.

Alcoholism rehabilitation treatment modalities have a heavy reliance on lecture style teaching and process oriented verbal groups. Experience has shown positive response to task and activity oriented occupational therapy groups. The value of occupational therapy intervention with alcoholics still needs to be proven.

REFERENCES

Agne, C., & Paolucci, K. (1982). A holistic health approach to an alcoholic treatment program. *Journal of Drug Education, 12*, 137-144.

Alcoholics Anonymous World Services, Inc. (1952). *Twelve steps and twelve traditions*. New York, NY: Author.

American Occupational Therapy Association. (1986). *Member data survey*. Rockville, MD: Author.

Bailey, M. B. (1970). Attitudes toward alcoholism before and after training program for social caseworkers. *Quarterly Journal for Studies on Alcohol, 31*, 669-683.

Barth, T. (1980). Occupational therapy services in alcoholism treatment. *Alcoholism/substance abuse information packet* (pp. 51-54). Rockville, MD: The American Occupational Therapy Association.

Buys, D., & Saltman, J. (1982). *The unseen alcoholics: The elderly*. (Public Affairs Pamphlet #602.) New York, NY: Public Affairs Committee.

Cassidy, C. L. (1985). [Occupational therapy education programs alcoholism instruction questionnaire.] Unpublished raw data.

Chappel, J. N., & Schnoll, S. H. (1977). Physicians' attitudes: Effects on the treatment of chemically dependent patients. *Journal of American Medical Association, 237*, 2318-2319.

DiCicco, L. M., & Unterberger, H. (1977). Cultural and professional avoidance: A dilemma in alcoholism training. *Journal of Alcohol and Drug Education, 22*, 28-38.

Dobie, J. (1978). *Substance abuse among the elderly*. Toronto, Canada: Addiction Research Foundation of Toronto.

Doniger, J. M. (1953). An activity program with alcoholics. *The American Journal of Occupational Therapy, 7*, 110-112, 135.

Dorsch, G., & Talley, R. (1973). Responses to alcoholics by the helping professions in Denver. *Quarterly Journal for Studies on Alcohol, 34*, 165-172.

Engelhardt, H. T. (1977). Defining occupational therapy: The meaning of therapy and the virtues of occupation. *The American Journal of Occupational Therapy, 31*, 666-672.

Fisher, J. C., Mason, R. L., Keeley, K. A., & Fisher, J. V. (1975). Physicians and alcoholics. *Journal of Studies on Alcohol, 36*, 949-955.

Hossack, J. R. (1952). Clinical trial of occupational therapy in the treatment of alcohol addiction. *The American Journal of Occupational Therapy, 6*, 265-266, 282.

Kinney, J., & Leaton, G. (1983). *Loosening the grip: A handbook of alcoholism information* (2nd ed.). St. Louis: The C. V. Mosby Company.

Kurtz, F. (1979). *Not God: A history of Alcoholics Anonymous*. Center City, MN: Hazelden Educational Services.

Larson, A. (1971). Occupational therapy study — 1969. *Canadian Journal of Occupational Therapy, 38*(3), 115-120.

Larson, A. (1971). Occupational therapy in a therapeutic milieu. *Canadian Journal of Occupational Therapy*, *38*(4), 156-162.

Lidz, T. (1966). Adolph Meyer and the development of American psychiatry. *American Journal of Psychiatry*, *123*, 320-332.

Lindsay, W. P. (1983). The role of the occupational therapist in the treatment of alcoholism. *The American Journal of Occupational Therapy*, *37*, 36-43.

Macdonald, E. M. (Ed.). (1976). *Occupational therapy in rehabilitation* (4th ed.). Baltimore: The Williams and Wilkins Company.

Maiorana, R. (1983). The role of the occupational therapist. *Alcoholism/substance abuse information packet* (p. 55). Rockville, MD: The American Occupational Therapy Association.

Marston, E. R. (1942). The use of occupational therapy in the treatment of alcoholics. *Occupational Therapy and Rehabilitation*, *21*, 350-352.

Meyer, A. (1922). The philosophy of occupational therapy. *Archives of Occupational Therapy*, *1*, 1-10.

Meyer, A. (1937, September). *In honor of Eleanor Clark Slagle*. Address presented at testimonial banquet, Atlantic City, NJ.

National Council on Alcoholism. (1982). Alcohol and alcoholism: Facts, figures and findings. (Available from Santa Clara County NCA, 1617 Willowhurst Avenue, San Jose, CA 95125.)

National Council on Alcoholism. (1983). Alcohol and teenagers fact sheet. (Available from Santa Clara County NCA.)

National Council on Alcoholism. (1981). No comment fact sheet. (Available from Santa Clara County NCA.)

National Institute on Alcohol Abuse and Alcoholism. (1981). *Fourth special report to the U.S. congress on alcohol and health*. (DHHS Publication No. ADM 81-1080.) Rockville, MD: U.S. Government Printing Office.

Shannon, P. D. (1972). Work-play theory and the occupational therapy process. *The American Journal of Occupational Therapy*, *26*, 169-172.

Smith, J. W. (1983). Diagnosing alcoholism. *Hospital and Community Psychiatry*, *34*, 1017-1021.

Smith, T. M., & Glickstein, C. S. (1980-81). Art as a therapeutic modality for individuals with alcohol-related problems in a milieu setting. *Occupational Therapy in Mental Health*, *1*, 33-43.

Welsh, J. (1959). Occupational therapy contributions in the treatment of the alcoholic. *The American Journal of Occupational Therapy*, *13*, 157-161, 176.

Weschler, H., & Rohman, M. (1982). Future caregivers' views on alcoholism treatment: A poor prognosis. *Journal of Studies on Alcohol*, *43*, 939-955.

Zimberg, S., Lipscomb, H., & David, E. B. (1971). Socio-psychiatric treatment of alcoholism in an urban ghetto. *American Journal of Psychiatry*, *127*, 106-110.

An Organizational Framework
for Occupational Therapy
in the Treatment of Alcoholism

Penelope A. Moyers, MS, OTR

SUMMARY. Because occupational therapists are increasingly involved with alcoholism rehabilitation, an organizational treatment framework is presented that is based upon the psychodynamics of this diagnosis. Factors that contribute to the development of a unique defense structure characteristic of alcoholism are discussed as prerequisites for understanding the treatment needs of the adult. Treatment is organized into three hierarchical levels that correspond with progressive changes in the alcoholics' defense structure. Alcoholics at level one require directive treatment approaches that do not aggressively confront the preferred, but maladaptive defense mechanisms in order to attain abstinence. Teaching coping strategies that provide alternatives to the preferred defense mechanisms are beneficial at level two. The third level involves stimulating the arrested emotional development of the alcoholic thus effectively challenging the continued utilization of these defense mechanisms. Specific occupational therapy methods and frames of reference are outlined that are appropriate for implementation at each treatment level.

INTRODUCTION

Until recently, occupational therapists have not been aware of their role in the treatment of alcoholism. In the past, therapists' case loads included alcoholism, but only as a secondary diagnosis, if it

Penelope A. Moyers is Assistant Professor, Department of Occupational Therapy, University of Indianapolis, 1400 East Hanna Avenue, Indianapolis, IN 46227.

The author would like to thank Cati Barrett, MS, OTR and Zona Weeks, PhD, OTR. Without their assistance, this manuscript would not have been completed.

27

was recognized as a treatment problem at all. Even today, health professionals continue to "deny" the role that alcohol abuse plays in depression and other psychiatric and medical diagnoses (McCabe, 1978); but, the facts are that 10 million adults and three million children abuse alcohol (Barchas, 1985).

Occupational therapists have not articulated treatment approaches within their existing frames of reference that address the core psychological issues of the alcoholic. Therefore, the purpose of this paper is to describe the psychodynamics of alcoholism as a foundation for occupational therapy intervention and to provide an organized framework for treatment on an inpatient or outpatient basis. Treatment is divided into three hierarchical levels according to the work of Zimberg, Wallace, and Blume (1985). The concept of *preferred defense structure* (PDS) described by Wallace (1985) is introduced and is incorporated into the levels.

PSYCHODYNAMICS

When considering possible psychological causes of alcoholism, one major question surfaces, whether or not an addictive personality is a prerequisite for developing alcoholism. The term *addictive personality* is used to describe the "impulsive, aggressive, overly emotional" behavior patterns of the alcoholic (Lawson, Peterson, & Lawson, 1983, p. 8). Current research examining the causes of alcoholism indicates that there is probably no premorbid addictive personality (Royce, 1981). Personality traits seem to occur more from the effect of prolonged drinking (Madsen, 1973). However, caution needs to be exercised before ruling out all possibilities for psychological causes. According to Royce, too great an emphasis on the physiological origins of alcoholism creates "grave errors in diagnosis" (1981, p. 143). Generally, it is accepted that psychological, sociocultural, and physiological factors interact together as determinants of alcoholism.

According to Zimberg (1985), it is theorized that a constellation of key defense mechanisms is formulated in childhood. The child's interactions with significant others seem to produce the "core conflict that must be recognized in therapy" (Zimberg, 1985, p. 5). This constellation is common for most alcoholics but is not thought of as resulting in an addictive personality. Types of childhood relationships that may have fostered the alcoholic's overdependence upon specific defense mechanisms will now be delineated. The complexity involved must be emphasized even though the psychodynamic processes are simplified here for purposes of discussion.

One such relationship involves overprotection in which the child is never really allowed to mature. More common that this overprotection pattern are those relationships revolving around the parents' own abuse of alcohol and drugs. In fact, most family studies have reported higher incidence of alcoholism among relatives of alcoholics than in the general population (Goodwin, 1978). Children of alcoholics probably inherit a genetic predisposition to alcoholism (Smith, 1982). In addition, there exists both a sociocultural and a psychological impact upon these children from their environments.

As a result of their environment, children of alcoholics may experience rejection early in life from the drinking parent or parents. Rejection can be in the form of constant criticism to the point of verbal and/or physical abuse; at the very least, the child may be ignored altogether. It is likely that children of alcoholic parents suffer from some form or neglect. Approximately 77% of the reported child neglect cases in a study by Spieker and Mouzakitis (cited in Lawson et al., 1983) were in families where at least one of the parents was alcoholic.

Often the eldest child in the family will experience role reversal with the parents (Fox, 1972). In other words, this child assumes adult responsibilities by taking care of the other children in the family as well as taking care of the drinking parent(s) (Cork, 1969). In the case where one parent is sober, involvement with his or her own emotional pain is so great that the effect of the drinking parent's behavior on the children is not noticed.

The dynamics produced by various childhood experiences involving an alcoholic parent may impede the child's emotional development if no intervention occurs (Chafetz, Blane, & Hill, 1971). Usually the child grows up experiencing unmet dependency needs (Blume, 1966). As an adult, need for nurturing leads this person to search for satisfying relationships; however, expectations of others are so unrealistic that this individual often believes that he or she is experiencing rejection.

Rejection from adult relationships arouses intense emotions of fear, anger, guilt, depression, and anxiety similar to the feelings experienced in childhood that were never consciously acknowledged. These feelings, related to fear of abandonment, create a need for compensation through the defense mechanisms of denial and grandiosity. The adult is convinced that nothing is wrong and that he or she is better than others. This grandiosity sets up a pattern of overwork either on the job or within relationships. Eventually this person experiences some kind of failure that triggers the same intense emotions.

If this person's cultural environment accepts alcohol in social use, and if this person biologically tolerates alcohol without too many adverse side-effects, it is likely that alcohol will be used as a coping method to escape from anxiety (Smith, 1982). The sedative effects reduce the intensity of anxiety, allowing denial and grandiosity to remain effective as compensation mechanisms. A repetitive cycle may begin that includes trying harder, experiencing failure, responding with intense feelings, compensating with denial or grandiosity, and coping through the use of alcohol. If uninterrupted, this cycle eventually leads to psychological dependency upon alcohol and, depending on the biological make-up, may lead to physiological dependency in the future (Zimberg, 1985).

The main point to remember in terms of psychodynamics is the possibility of impaired emotional development and unmet dependency needs in the alcoholic (McCord & McCord, 1960). Use of alcohol allows the escape from intense emotions evoked by situations that fail to provide security and reassure abandonment fears.

PREFERRED DEFENSE STRUCTURE

According to Wallace, one of several preferred defense structures (PDS) is developed and utilized by the alcoholic (1985). This PDS may be defined as "a collection of skills or abilities, tactics and strategies, for achieving one's ends" that have been learned and integrated into daily modes of behavior (Wallace, 1985, p. 26). These defense structures are based upon the psychodynamics previously described. Without understanding the individual's PDS, professionals may find themselves engaged in counter-transference in response to the alcoholic's behavior elicited in treatment. Perhaps this lack of understanding contributed to earlier beliefs that alcoholics were basically not treatable (Douglass, 1976).

The possibility that during childhood the alcoholic learned to use specific defense mechanisms to avoid feelings needs to be reemphasized. While actively drinking as an adult, this unique defense structure is further developed and modified to accomplish that same objective. The typical response of the health professional when encountering this defense structure is to confront the alcoholic. The professional may not realize that confrontation creates intense, reactionary feelings within the alcoholic. Such feelings prompt that pattern of coping involving denial, grandiosity, and drinking to escape. If the alcoholic is not ready for confrontation, then the urge to drink will intensify, making it difficult to stay in treatment.

Instead, Wallace (1985) advocates that the PDS not be removed totally, at least initially, but be mobilized toward the goal of maintaining abstinence. Only that part of the PDS that inhibits abstinence is confronted. The alcoholic is not stripped of the only method of coping he or she knows before it can be replaced through treatment with alternative, more healthy strategies.

The following is a discussion of the major defense mechanisms that make up the PDS. Some review is included regarding the defense mechanism's function in allowing the alcoholic to avoid feelings and to continue drinking; however, the process of mobilizing the defense structure as a part of treatment by occupational therapists will be highlighted.

Denial

The most important aspect of the PDS is denial (Wallace, 1985). This defense mechanism has already played a major role in avoiding the core conflict developed in childhood, i.e., unmet dependency needs. It is logical to assume that when drinking, the role of denial becomes even more important. Denial is also notorious for its prevalence in the alcoholic's behavior, and many people are aware that denial is one of the symptoms of alcoholism used in making the diagnosis (Zimberg, 1982).

Basically, denial promotes continued drinking and the ignoring of issues regardless of mounting evidence that problems are increasing and that drinking is actually part of the problem. Denial, then, is usually thought of as something bad and becomes the immediate focus of treatment. But, in the professionals' zeal to get the alcoholic to admit to being addicted and to face problems, the alcoholic becomes overwhelmed and may feel hopeless. At this point, abstinence cannot be maintained. The feelings are too intense and the alcoholic "has to drink."

The alternative is to let the alcoholic believe for a time that the problems result from drinking even though not all of them do. Eventually, realization occurs that some problems will continue to exist during sobriety. The occupational therapist's role is to assist problem solving concerning only those issues related to drinking. Problems as a result of the alcoholic's personality and immature emotional development are not dealt with initially. The therapist utilizes structured, concrete activities that avoid premature self-disclosure. Uncovering techniques such as expressive media are not employed in the beginning of treatment.

Projection

After denial, projection is probably next in terms of importance (Blume, 1966). The alcoholic's own feelings are attributed to others, not only to avoid feelings but to maintain excuses regarding the need to drink. One of the best "reasons" to drink involves the belief that people who are important in the alcoholic's life are angry with the alcoholic. The person involved may not be angry or even be aware of the alcoholic's attitude.

Occupational therapists can respond by encouraging reality testing regarding the alcoholic's perceptions of feelings held by others. Most important, however, is using projection to promote treatment. Wallace describes *assimilative projection* (1985, p. 28), which means the alcoholic learns that he or she is like other alcoholics because of having similar feelings and experiences. There is a sense of relief in discovering that others face the same predicaments. The occupational therapist capitalizes on assimilative projection by planning group activities that develop trust and foster the feeling of mutual respect. Competitive-type group activities are not used initially.

Rationalization

This defense mechanism provides the alcoholic with seemingly logical reasons for drinking. Rationalizations are exceptionally resistant to confrontation. The therapist should remember that the function of rationalization is to avoid painful reality (Blume, 1966). Because reality, if faced too soon, can perpetuate a need to drink that results in leaving treatment, rationalization becomes a useful tool to maintain sobriety. Pain can be avoided until the person is adequately prepared for it. In a way, it can be said that the alcoholic rationalizes why he or she needs to be sober. Reasons to stay sober, as "my boss might fire me" or "my wife might leave me," are some prime examples.

The occupational therapist can employ *sober rationalization* in the beginning stages of treatment (Wallace, 1985, p. 30). This is done by having the alcoholic identify the sociocultural problems he or she is currently experiencing (poor job performance, school failure, or difficulty socializing, etc.), and the part drinking had in aggravating these problems. Often, the alcoholic willingly commits to changing these problem areas before working through the major issues of the addiction.

Dichotomous Thinking

The alcoholic may have experienced uncertainty in the past as a result of a chaotic family structure. As a child, an alcoholic may have had parents who displayed unpredictable, alcoholic behavior. The alcoholic learned to compensate by preferring certainty and as a result became intolerant of the "gray areas." This restricted alternatives available in problem solving and created judgmental attitudes (Wallace, 1985). The occupational therapist can utilize this desire for predictability by providing a unit schedule as well as involving the alcoholic in structured groups, well-planned individual sessions, and organized social situations.

The occupational therapist also must guard against certain critical issues based upon this preference for dichotomous thinking from

being evoked by the intervention itself. Treatment methods that in-
advertently produce denial of the alcoholism, such as by excessively focusing on sociocultural problems (e.g., financial or marital
problems) are as detrimental as those that promote premature self-
disclosure. Facing guilt too quickly because of intense confrontation or avoiding accepting a "normal" amount of guilt because of
too great an emphasis upon the disease concept of alcoholism by the
therapist is another dichotomy that can occur.

Other examples of this tendency for "all-or-none" thinking are:
engaging in excessive self-blaming or blaming others, rebelling
against rules or becoming overly compliant, impulsively expressing
feelings by acting out or repressing feelings, focusing obsessively
on the past or refusing to explore it, becoming overly dependent
upon staff and peers or refusing to accept help, compulsively socializing or withdrawing, demonstrating perfectionism or disregarding
quality of performance, exhibiting narcissism or focusing totally on
others, and acting either pessimistic or overly optimistic (Wallace,
1985).

The occupational therapist designs experiences that promote safe
exploration of the middle ground in each of these dichotomous issues. In effect, the repertoire of behavioral alternatives necessary
for responding appropriately to everyday situations is enlarged. For
example, an alcoholic involved in a craft group may in one session
exhibit too much attention to detail and the next time may carelessly
proceed through the task steps. Initially, the therapist assists the
alcoholic in deciding when imperfections are to be tolerated and
when they are not to be tolerated. It is in the later stages of treatment that the therapist encouraged the examination of how these
behaviors have been utilized in the past to avoid complex issues and
feelings.

TREATMENT LEVELS

As implied throughout the previous discussion, treatment is implemented according to three hierarchical levels which are organized to reflect progressive changes in the PDS as the alcoholic
recovers (Zimberg, 1985). Table 1 summarizes each treatment level
by outlining the corresponding PDS status, treatment issue, treat-

Table 1
Treatment Levels

Treatment Levels	PDS Status	Treatment Issue	Treatment Setting	Roles		
				Alcoholic	Family	Treatment Team
1	Mobilized	Abstinence	Inpatient	Accept External Control	Alanon Alcohol/Drug Education	Detoxification Alcohol/Drug Education Nutrition Rest Antabase AA/Alanon Milieu Directive Psychotherapy
2	Weakened	Coping Strategies	Inpatient or Outpatient	Develop Internal Control	Alanon Family Therapy	Directive Psychotherapy Supportive Psychotherapy AA/Alanon Milieu Family Therapy
3	Confronted	Emotional Development	Outpatient or Extended Treatment	Relate Maturely	Alanon Psychodynamic Family Therapy	Psychodynamic Psychotherapy AA/Alanon Family Therapy

ment setting, and role of the alcoholic, family, and treatment team. Refer to this table throughout the following discussion. The role of the occupational therapist will be discussed in a later section.

In the first level of treatment, usually provided on an inpatient basis, the focus is on abstinence and the alcoholic's role is one of accepting external control for the drinking. The PDS is not challenged, but is mobilized to assist in maintaining abstinence. Level one usually corresponds with the detoxification process. The role of the treatment team and family is one of providing the external control. This is accomplished through detoxification, alcohol/drug education, nutrition, rest, Antabuse, directive psychotherapy, Alcoholic's Anonymous (AA), Alanon, and the treatment milieu (Zimberg, 1985).

Treatment emphasis at level two is upon developing healthier coping strategies and may either occur on an inpatient or outpatient basis. Detoxification by this time has been completed, unless complications have resulted. Permanent brain damage secondary to long-term use of alcohol may be severe enough to prevent progression to this treatment level and the following third level.

During level-two treatment, the PDS weakens as the alcoholic learns these alternative coping strategies and starts to "prefer" them over drinking. Gradually, external control is being replaced by the alcoholic's newly emerging ability to maintain abstinence through internal control. The treatment team provides some directive psychotherapy, but this eventually transforms into supportive psychotherapy (Zimberg, 1985). AA is continued and the alcoholic is encouraged to assume a leadership role in the treatment milieu. The family continues to attend Alanon and now is involved in family therapy with the alcoholic.

Level three intervention can be thought of as stimulating the alcoholic's emotional development. This occurs usually on an outpatient basis if treatment was successful, or in an extended treatment situation if more intensive therapy is required. Very rarely does this occur during the initial inpatient hospitalization. It is at this level that the PDS is finally thoroughly confronted and by the alcoholic's choice "given up." If the alcoholic does not choose to give up the PDS, long-term sobriety is threatened. Therefore, programs that do not include this level of treatment may not have as low a recidivism rate as those that do include this aspect (Royce, 1981).

The alcoholic's role in treatment is to continue attending AA, to relate to others maturely, and to begin the process of introspection. The family remains in Alanon and attends family therapy along with the alcoholic. Family therapy is more psychodynamically oriented, as is the alcoholic's individual and group psychotherapy (Zimberg, 1985).

TREATMENT LEVELS AND OCCUPATIONAL THERAPY

These three treatment levels can serve as an organizing framework for occupational therapy intervention. The framework assists in selecting the most appropriate frame of reference for guiding each patient's evaluation, treatment planning, treatment implementation, and treatment evaluation processes. Utilizing the concept of treatment levels ensures that the alcoholic's PDS status is considered when making the selection. In this way, the choice is based upon the current treatment issue, i.e., whether the alcoholic requires external control in order to attain abstinence, the teaching of coping strategies in order to foster internal control, or the stimulation of emotional development in order to maintain long-term sobriety.

The frame of reference selection process is addressed by focusing on seven frames of reference used in occupational therapy. These seven include: (1) Management of Cognitive Disabilities, (2) Behavioral, (3) Recapitulation of Ontogenesis, (4) Model of Human Occupation, (5) Biomechanical, (6) Cognitive-behavioral, and (7) Object Relations. This discussion is not meant to provide a review of the details of these frames of reference. It does provide an analysis and a sense of which frame of reference appears to be the most applicable to specific patient problems common at each treatment level. The ability of each frame of reference to address the PDS status and corresponding treatment issue at the particular level is given priority in the discussion. Refer to Tables 2 through 4 in order to discern usage of these seven frames of reference at each treatment level.

It is this author's contention that no one frame of reference is

Table 2
Level 1 and Occupational Therapy

Problems

Frame of Reference	Cognitive	Physical Daily Living	Sensorimotor	Psychosocial	Psychological
Management of Cognitive Disabilities	Task analysis Semistandardized tasks	Routine tasks	N/A	Structured environment	Successful task experience
Model of Human Occupation	Process skill development	Self-care skill development Self-care habits	Perceptual-motor skill development	Communication/Interaction skill development	Development of personal causation Exploration of interests and values
Behavioral	N/A	Reinforcement Shaping, chaining Modeling Privileges Token economies	Biofeedback Desensitization Repetition Reinforcement	Reinforcement Modeling Role Playing	N/A
Recapitulation of Ontogenesis	Cognitive skill	N/A	Perceptual-motor skill	Dyadic-interaction skill	Drive-object skill
Biomechanical	N/A	Remediation Adaptation Compensation	Physical endurance Coordination Strengthening	N/A	Satisfaction from improved physical performance

PDS Status: Mobilized
Treatment Issue: Abstinence

Table 3
Level 2 and Occupational Therapy

Problems

	Psychological	Psycho-Social	Work	Leisure	Prevention
Cognitive-Behavioral	Rational-emotive therapy Beck's cognitive therapy	Assertiveness training	Assertiveness training Stress management Psycho-educational groups	Stress management	Stress management Psychoeducational groups Evaluating the person-environment match Discharge planning
Behavioral	N/A	Structured-learning therapy Modeling Role Playing Reinforcement	Prevocational & vocational training Modeling Role Playing Reinforcement	Avocational training Modeling Reinforcement	Biofeedback Determining environmental demands for behavior Transfer of training Fieldtrips Discharge planning
Model of Human Occupation	Competence Level of: Interest identification Personal causation values	Reestablishing social roles & habits Competence & achievement levels of communication/interaction skills	Reestablishing existing work roles & work habits Time management	Reestablishing leisure habits Engaging in identified interests Time management	Determining environmental support for change (physical & social) Fieldtrips Discharge planning
Recapitulation of Ontogenesis	N/A	Group interaction skills	N/A	N/A	N/A

PDS Status: Weakened
Treatment Issue: Coping Strategies

Table 4
Level 3 and Occupational Therapy

Problems

Psychological: Self-awareness, self-identity, self-expression, & self-actualization

Object Relations	Symbol production Identification of needs Exploration of the unconscious Creative expression Group process
Recapitulation of Ontogenesis	Sexual identity skill development Self-identity skill development
Model of Human Occupation	Achievement level: previous values, interests, personal causation, roles, habits, and skills Exploratory level of new values and interests Establishing new roles and habits Developing new, complex skills

PDS Status: Confronted
Treatment Issue: Emotional development

useful for the treatment of all alcoholics across treatment levels. When employing a single frame of reference, according to Bruce and Borg, "it is not just the lack of rigorous and broad empirical evidence, but it is also the denial of individual difference and the limitation of individual preference and option that is a concern" (1987, p. 349). Because treatment emphasis changes as the alcoholic progresses through the three levels, it is found that some frames of reference address these issues better than others. Finally, the fact that the treatment levels integrate inpatient and outpatient therapy over a period of several years necessitates that frames of reference correspond to the therapist involved, facility, and setting.

Occupational therapists, as shown in Table 2, help level-one alcoholics by conducting cognitive, sensorimotor, psychosocial, psychological, and physical daily living skills evaluations and indicated treatment. As the alcoholic's thinking clears and withdrawal symptoms lessen, the therapist monitors and reports cognitive, physical, and behavioral improvements reflected by performance. One of several frames of reference is useful, depending upon the alcoholic's needs and the existence of any residual organic or physical deficits.

For example, if cognition, i.e., orientation, conceptualization, comprehension, or integration is a major problem area, Allen's frame of reference, Management of Cognitive Disabilities, may be utilized (1985). Because of the attention that this frame of reference gives to structuring the external environment, it fulfills the level-one criteria of providing external control. Also, through periodic cognitive-level evaluation, the detoxification process can be monitored by involving the alcoholic in routine tasks and semistandardized tasks (Allen, 1985). If permanent cognitive impairment appears likely, the occupational therapist can provide information concerning the alcoholic's ability to live independently. In addition, the therapist can offer consultation to team members regarding adaptation of the treatment program components that traditionally require intact cognitive capacities in order to participate, e.g., family and group therapy.

There are other frames of reference that address cognition, but to a lesser degree, such as The Model of Human Occupation (process skills) and Recapitulation of Ontogenesis (cognitive skill). The strength of these frames of reference lies in the ability to deal with a variety of problems that are treated at level one other than cognition of which impaired psychosocial functioning and sensorimotor deficits are examples.

Another feature is the potential usefulness of these two frames of reference during the next treatment levels. Management of Cognitive Disabilities is not theoretically effective at levels two and three as it makes little, if any, provisions for promoting internal control and stimulating emotional development. Preventing any difficulties that might result when switching from one frame of reference to another with the same patient is an important consideration. Therefore, if cognition seems to be a temporary deficit, perhaps one of the other frames of reference should be selected. For instance, if psychosocial performance is determined to be the emphasis for treatment at level one, the behavioral frame of reference describes modeling, reinforcement, and role playing as methods to change maladaptive behavior to more adaptive behavior (Bruce & Borg, 1987).

Due to the level-one requirement for the therapist to provide external control, it is obvious that the object relations frame of reference should not be chosen. Many of the activities utilized within this frame of reference are unstructured so that projection of the patient's needs and feelings onto the activity itself may occur. Developing insight is the goal of the Object Relations frame of reference resulting in PDS confrontation which should not happen until level three (Bruce & Borg, 1987). This violates the concept of mobilizing the existing PDS. The most beneficial frames of reference lend themselves to effective use of denial, sober rationalizations, assimilative projection, and expansion of the behavioral repertoire from the restricted, dichotomous form of thinking and acting.

Therefore, it follows that level-one approaches within a particular frame of reference should include structured tasks that utilize successful experiences as a means to satisfy unmet dependency needs. The therapist plans the treatment sessions with the alcoholic's input but has primary responsibility for their organization. Group activities are essentially noncompetitive in nature, building trust and rapport among the group's members. Treatment sessions help the alcoholic determine the relationship between drinking and life problems, such as poor job performance or school failure. Reestablishing normal routines, especially physical daily living habits and social roles, is important. If physical complications are evident, the biomechanical frame of reference may be employed. Craft groups, ADL groups, reality orientation, mild exercise, and task groups are examples of approaches offered for level-one alcoholics within these frames of reference. Other groups might include problem identification, socialization, communication, and social skills.

Occupational therapy at level two involves teaching alternative coping and prevention strategies. Family members may be involved along with the alcoholic so that they can also learn these coping strategies and prevention techniques. Within a cognitive-behavioral frame of reference, assertiveness training, stress management, rational-emotive therapy and other psychoeducational groups are useful (Bruce & Borg, 1987). Typical patient problems dealt with by groups at the second level include psychological, psychosocial, work, and leisure impairments. (See Table 3.)

Groups that are concerned with lifestyle adjustment (as time management and leisure counseling) are appropriate. Work skills such as homemaking, parenting, and employment preparation are addressed. Physical exercise through games and sports that are more competitive may be utilized. Field trips to the community expose the alcoholic and the family to possible support systems that may be utilized in the future to promote continued, independent coping. Transfer of skills from hospital to home is thus more likely to occur. These groups may be conducted within the Model of Human Occupation or a behavioral frame of reference.

Regardless of the occupational therapy frame of reference and implementation methods chosen at level two, the alcoholic and the family are given more responsibility in selecting, planning, and implementing activities. The therapist also promotes independent rehearsal of these coping strategies by asking the alcoholic and family members to try out new skills in other therapy groups, during family therapy, within the treatment milieu, and during AA/Alanon meetings. Results of these efforts are shared in the occupational therapy sessions. In addition, the alcoholic and the family, with the therapist's guidance, develop a discharge plan that structures coping alternatives into a daily schedule to be followed at home. Appropriate outlets for emotion are fostered so that they become a part of the alcoholic's and the family's lifestyle. Discharge planning groups are effective in accomplishing these objectives and preventing unnecessary rehospitalizations because of lack of follow-through.

At level three, the occupational therapist promotes self-awareness, self-identity, self-expression, and self-actualization. This is accomplished through group, individual, or family sessions that utilize projective and expressive techniques. Developing insight is a major goal, and because of this, the object relations frame of reference is compatible. Group implementation methods for the object relations frame of reference may include needs identification through group processing and creative symbol production to explore the unconscious. However, the Recapitulation of Ontogenesis frame of reference may be selected if the focus is on developing only self-identity and sexual identity skills (Bruce & Borg, 1987). (See Table 4.)

Usually, self-analysis and self-discovery lead to new risk-taking behaviors. The therapist may need to guide the alcoholic, and when appropriate, family members through problem solving centered around these new life experiences. It could be the first time in many years that personal decisions related to career and family or other interpersonal relationships are made maturely. In this respect, the Model of Human Occupation is helpful as it ensures that old values corrupted by the drinking process are reestablished and that unfamiliar values are explored (Kielhofner, 1985). New goals, interests, roles, and skills for the future are determined based upon these values, and a deeper sense of personal causation is achieved. Values clarification groups and problem solving groups are examples of the program offered at treatment level three within this frame of reference.

Specific to this treatment level and regardless of the frame of reference employed, the alcoholic performs most of the therapeutic activities on his or her own outside of the formal group sessions. This is necessary because level three treatment primarily is part of outpatient programs and occurs usually during the final phase of treatment. The therapist and other group members assist in selecting the therapeutic task and monitor results by requiring evidence of actual implementation and feedback regarding the outcomes. In this way, the alcoholic is held responsible for his or her own emotional development and any dependency upon professionals is discouraged.

CONCLUSION

Currently, intervention within the existing occupational therapy frames of reference is often implemented without regard to the unique, underlying psychodynamics of the alcoholic individual. It is important for the therapist to understand the preferred defense structure at each of the three proposed treatment levels. Because of this understanding, the occupational therapist can select the most appropriate frame of reference that is compatible with each level's treatment issue and the patient's particular problems.

At level one, an external source of control should be provided that mobilizes the alcoholic's PDS. Coping strategies that weaken the PDS should be taught at level two. Finally, at level three, emotional development should be stimulated in order to confront continued usage of the PDS by the alcoholic. From a variety of approaches and frames of reference used in occupational therapy, a suitable treatment program for these three levels and their specific treatment concerns can be developed. Thus, occupational therapy can be an asset to the overall treatment program conducted in acute inpatient and outpatient, or long-term inpatient treatment facilities.

REFERENCES

Allen, C. K. (1985). *Occupational therapy for psychiatric diseases: Measurement and management of cognitive disabilities*. Boston: Little, Brown and Company.

Barchas, J. D. (1985). Research on mental illness and addictive disorders. *American Journal of Psychiatry, 142*(7) (Supplement, July).

Blume, E. M. (1966). Psychoanalytic views of alcoholism: A review. *Quarterly Journal of Studies on Alcohol, 27*, 259-299.

Bruce, M. A., & Borg, B. (1987). *Frames of reference in psychosocial occupational therapy*. New Jersey: Slack.

Chafetz, M. E., Blane, H. T., & Hill, M. J. (1971). Children of alcoholics: Observations in a child guidance clinic. *Quarterly Journal of Studies on Alcohol, 32*, 687-689.

Cork, M. R. (1969). *The forgotten children*. Toronto: Paperjacks, in association with Addiction Research Foundation.

Douglas, D. B. (1976). Who is a real alcoholic? Practical help in managing alcoholism. *New York State Journal of Medicine*, 76, 603-607.

Fox, R. (1972). *The effect of alcoholism on children*. New York: National Council on Alcoholism.

Goodwin, D. W. (1978). The genetics of alcoholism: A state of the art review. *Alcohol Health and Research World*, 2, 2-12.

Kielhofner, G. (Ed.). (1985). *A model of human occupation: Theory and application*. Baltimore: Williams and Wilkins.

Lawson, G., Peterson, J. S., & Lawson, A. (1983). *Alcoholism and the family*. Rockville, MD: Aspen.

Madsen, W. (1973). *The American alcoholic: The nature-nurture controversy in alcoholic research*. Springfield, IL: Charles C Thomas.

McCabe, T. R. (1978). *Victims no more*. Center City, MN: Hazelden.

McCord, W., & McCord, J. (1960). *Origins of alcoholism*. Stanford: Stanford University Press.

Royce, J. E. (1981). *Alcohol problems and alcoholism: A comprehensive survey*. New York: Macmillan.

Smith, M. (1982). The genetics of alcoholism. In B. Stimmel (Ed.), *The effects of maternal alcohol and drug abuse on the newborn* (pp. 127-145). New York: The Haworth Press, Inc.

Wallace, J. (1985). Working with the preferred defense structure of the recovering alcoholic. In S. Zimberg, J. Wallace, & S. Blume (Eds.), *Practical approaches to alcoholism psychotherapy* (2nd ed.) (pp. 23-35). New York: Plenum Press.

Zimberg, S. (1982). *The clinical management of alcoholism*. New York: Brunner/Mazel.

Zimberg, S., Wallace, J., & Blume, S. B. (1985). *Practical approaches to alcoholism psychotherapy* (2nd ed.). New York: Plenum Press.

Zimberg, S. (1985). Principles of alcoholism psychotherapy. In S. Zimberg, J. Wallace, & S. Blume (Eds.), *Practical approaches to alcoholism psychotherapy* (2nd ed.) (pp. 3-22). New York: Plenum Press.

Abstinence-Oriented Inpatient Treatment of the Substance Abuser

Jeffrey M. Klein, PhD

SUMMARY. Clinical issues related to the treatment of chemical dependency are delineated. The desirability of abstinence from all mood-altering drugs for the addict, and the view of chemical dependency as a primary illness rather than an underlying symptom are examined. A specific inpatient chemical dependency treatment program is described. In this treatment program, an interdisciplinary approach is employed which individualizes treatment goals to break through the patient's denial. In addition to the person's learning about the illness of chemical dependency and the effect that it has had on his functioning, the individual learns skills to facilitate interpersonal and psychological coping and growth. The role of occupational therapy in such a treatment setting is also highlighted.

Although the news media has heightened general awareness concerning the seriousness of drug usage and drug addiction, relatively little attention has been given to how mental health professionals actually treat the chemically dependent individual once this problem has been identified. This article will focus on various aspects of the theoretical and pragmatic issues related to inpatient drug treatment.

Jeffrey M. Klein is Chief of Service, Chemical Dependency Treatment Unit, Sheppard Pratt Hospital, 6501 N. Charles Street, Towson, MD 21204.

47

PHILOSOPHY AND MISSION

Several theoretical issues must be raised to highlight certain key controversies in the field of chemical dependency treatment: (1) methadone maintenance versus abstinence-oriented treatment; (2) "controlled" alcohol and drug usage versus an abstinence-oriented perspective; (3) chemical dependency versus addiction to specific chemical substances; and (4) chemical dependency as a "primary illness" rather than a symptom of underlying pathology.

Methadone Maintenance versus Abstinence-Oriented Treatment

Much of the early literature on the treatment of chemical dependency has focused on methadone maintenance treatment. For the most part, problems concerning addiction were often equated to narcotic and opiate addiction, whereas problems concerning the abuse of marijuana, cocaine and tranquilizers were not given a great deal of attention. It was felt that individuals with opiate addictions were not able to remain drug-free and, at best, the individual's functioning could be stabilized by providing a legally obtainable opiate such as methadone. By providing methadone, the addict would not need to obtain drugs illegally and engage in a variety of illegal activities to pay for drugs. As a result, the addict would be able to maintain stable family and work functioning and remain out of jail. Although this approach has been beneficial to some, it did not turn out to be the panacea it was originally hoped to be (Dole and Nyswander, 1976; Bratter, Pennacchia, and Gauya, 1985).

Recently, more treatment programs have begun to focus on the possibility of developing a new drug-free lifestyle using self-help groups as a source of support and encouragement. This type of treatment approach, which was adapted from alcohol treatment models, is not only geared to help the person become totally free of mood-altering drugs. In addition, the addict is taught new attitudes, new skills and new behaviors that would facilitate drug-free functioning and improve the addict's ability to cope with the tasks of daily living (Klein and Miller, 1986).

"Controlled" Alcohol and Drug Usage versus Abstinence-Oriented Perspectives

In the 1960s and 1970s, cognitive behavioral psychologists maintained that alcohol and drug problems can be viewed as learned behaviors; therefore it was felt that individuals should be taught to moderate their drug and alcohol intake. Using various cognitive and behavioral techniques, chemically dependent individuals were taught new skills to attempt to keep their alcohol and drug consumption at an acceptably "controlled" level (Marlott, 1978).

However, many individuals in the drug and alcohol treatment field believe that individuals with chemical dependency problems need to be totally drug-free. One of the rationales for such an approach comes from Alcoholics Anonymous. This organization maintains that alcohol and drug addiction is a chronic progressive illness that cannot be cured but can be arrested by means of abstinence from mood-altering substances (Narcotics Anonymous Big Book, 1984).

Others arrived at this abstinence-oriented view on the basis of recent psychological biochemical medical research. Milam and Ketcham (1983) for example postulated that biological triggers exist in the chemically dependent individual that make it less likely that alcohol usage can be stopped or moderated. Since "willpower" or determination cannot suitably counteract these biological mechanisms, two individuals who have used the same amount of a given mood-altering substance might react in a totally different fashion. This mechanism regarding alcohol consumption appears to be related to how alcohol is metabolized in the body, and drug addiction is hypothesized to have similar metabolic types of triggers. It is therefore not seen as a matter of psychological or moral weakness, but a complex interaction of biochemistry, genetics and exposure to mood-altering substances.

The Concept of Chemical Dependency versus the Notion of Addiction to a Specific Drug or Substance

There is some disagreement in the drug treatment field as to whether an individual who abuses *one* substance needs to be abstinent from other mood-altering chemicals. For example, does the cocaine abuser need to abstain from marijuana? Does the alcoholic need to be cautious about the use of tranquilizers? Does a heroin addict need to abstain from alcohol? Obviously each class of drug such as opiates, sedatives, amphetamines, etc. has a different chemical action on the body. There is little physiological data to conclusively indicate why it would be a problem for a heroin addict to drink alcohol since heroin and alcohol act so differently on physiological body processes. Nonetheless, those treating chemical dependency often find that two different patterns occur.

The first pattern involves the substitution of another class of drug for that originally used. Some individuals will stop using the particular drug that has effected them most adversely, but begin to use another substance which is seen as more innocuous. For example, an individual becomes cocaine-free, but begins drinking excessively because alcohol is seen as legal, cheaper, less problematic and less stigmatized.

A second more frequent pattern involves the disinhibition of the individual's "control" or vigilance that occurs as a result of the use of any mood-altering drug. As the individual's vigilance decreases and his mood is significantly altered he may be more susceptible to returning to the "high" of his favorite drug. It is not exactly clear how the psychological and physiological components combine to produce this disinhibition. Nonetheless, this phenomenon occurs often enough that many professionals believe that any substance abusing individual should remain free of all mood-altering drugs including alcohol.

Chemical Dependency as a Primary Illness Rather Than Merely a Symptom of Underlying Pathology

Some professionals, particularly those taking a psychodynamic view of substance abuse, focus on alcohol and drug problems as symptomatic of underlying psychological pathology. For example, they typically see drug abuse as an outgrowth of the individual's depression or his severe characterological impairment (Forrest, 1985). Although it is certainly true that individuals who are chemically dependent are not immune to affective or characterological disorders, many treatment professionals feel that it would be inaccurate to view chemical dependency as generally caused by such psychiatric issues. These professionals feel that as the individual becomes more and more impaired by the increasing use and abuse of chemicals, his functioning will become significantly impaired secondary to this drug abuse. This marked decrement in functioning would be likely to *produce* anxiety, dysphoria, depression, as well as impaired interpersonal, vocational and family functioning. Drug abuse and addiction may mimic, produce or magnify psychiatric disorder rather than addiction always being secondary to such dysfunction.

TREATMENT OPTIONS

In terms of treatment, the theoretical position taken on the four issues delineated previously will lead to very different routes for rehabilitation and treatment. For example, if the addiction is seen as secondary to an underlying psychiatric disorder, treatment would focus primarily on the patient's depression or characterological issues. From this perspective, drug usage will diminish as the true source of the problem is adequately dealt with and resolved. In contrast, those who view the addiction as a primary illness in and of itself, maintain that the key to treatment involves confronting the individual's denial and minimization of the seriousness and the danger of the progressive addictive illness. Only after the individual acknowledges the impact that substance abuse has had on his functioning will he begin to invest the energy to make changes in his alcohol and drug consumption as well as his general lifestyle.

Chemical Dependency Treatment Unit

After providing an overview of the wide range of professional perspectives and assumptions it is useful to examine one particular type of treatment program. The Chemical Dependency Treatment Unit at the Sheppard and Enoch Pratt Hospital in Baltimore, Maryland is an inpatient substance abuse unit advocating abstinence from all mood-altering drugs. The program's philosophies are heavily based on the principles of Narcotics Anonymous and Alcoholics Anonymous.

Patient Population

The Chemical Dependency Treatment Unit (CDTU) is a 13-bed adult short-term unit in a private psychiatric hospital. Sheppard Pratt also has a 15-bed inpatient unit that primarily treats individuals who abuse alcohol and sedatives. In contrast to that unit, the CDTU tends to treat drug abusers who are somewhat younger, more invested in a drug-related lifestyle, and who have more criminal or antisocial involvement. The tone of the CDTU is more confronting and more geared to deal with the maladaptive and deceptive style of this more antisocial population.

The length of stay on the inpatient treatment program is approximately 4 to 6 weeks. Individuals finance the treatment either through third party payment or private funds. The patient population tends to fall between 18 and 40 years of age and those who are older are typically treated on the other chemical dependency unit. Both males and females are treated, although the majority of patients have traditionally been men. Individuals on the CDTU have used a variety of drugs including cocaine, amphetamines, sedatives, opiates, alcohol, marijuana, PCP, and hallucinogens. Some are intravenous needle users. Some have been seriously abusing narcotics which have been prescribed for chronic pain.

Not all individuals need and/or can afford inpatient treatment of their chemical dependency. Depending on the frequency and pattern of drug usage, the need for inpatient detoxification, available support systems and psychiatric and characterological considerations, it may be possible for the patient to be treated on an outpatient basis. Although outpatient treatment is certainly a less disruptive and less expensive intervention, many individuals find it difficult to remain drug-free without a brief period of time outside the environment in which they were actively using drugs. A consultation with a mental health professional who is experienced in assessing chemical dependency problems can be useful in suggesting treatment options for the individual and his family.

Program Elements

This comprehensive and multidisciplinary program consists of several elements: (1) alcohol and drug education; (2) drug therapy groups focusing on the "First Step" (from Alcoholics Anonymous and Narcotics Anonymous); (3) teaching specific tools for recovery and skills that would facilitate living sober and drug-free; (4) individual psychotherapy and counseling; (5) family meetings and the family education program; (6) active participation in the Narcotics Anonymous and Alcoholics Anonymous Fellowship.

The most effective treatment modality for addiction is group therapy. Groups provide both the confrontation and the support that promotes honesty, decreases manipulation, deception, and distortion, and groups provide hope, encouragement, and role modeling for the recovery process. Furthermore, the individual's increased comfort in a group setting tends to facilitate his involvement with and participation in NA and AA Fellowships.

Although all chemically dependent patients are dealing with the same "disease," each individual has his unique life history, family constellation, and specific psychological and characterological issues. The present program tailors individualized treatment goals to address these specific cases. The treatment team's expectations of the patient's progress are based on the individual's particular cognitive and emotional strengths and weaknesses, the family and the vocational situation, the patient's previous treatment attempts, and the individual's drug and alcohol history. The most effective way to help the individual acknowledge the severity of his illness is to help him specify in detail how *his* drug and alcohol usage and the compulsivity of this behavior has adversely affected all aspects of *his* life. The individual begins to feel more hopeful as he gradually learns to cope with the specific situation he must face when he leaves the program.

1. Alcohol and Drug Education

The patient receives much information about the effects of the use and abuse of alcohol and mood-altering drugs on the mind, body and emotions of the substance abuser. Effects of the addiction on the mood behavior and attitude of the individual is carefully examined. Many substance abusers believe that they are "bad," "weak" or "stupid" because of their drug-related behaviors and their many failures and losses secondary to the progression of their illness. In these educational programs and discussions, the substance abuser learns that these patterns are created and/or greatly magnified by his drug usage. The individual begins to acknowledge that these past behaviors may not have to be seen in a harsh judgmental manner. Nonetheless, although the addict is not blamed for his being chemically dependent he needs to become more responsible in dealing with and treating his illness. Merely stating that his actions are a result of his addiction is not enough. He needs to learn how to "arrest this illness" and begin to take clear steps to develop a recovery program that will accomplish this.

2. Therapy Groups

These groups focus on helping the individual become more able to acknowledge the seriousness of his illness. The addict tends to see himself as "in control" and tends to see others as overreacting to his drug usage or drug-related behaviors. Since the addict does not see his situation as serious or "out of hand," he is not likely to put much energy into learning the behaviors necessary to change his lifestyle. To the extent the individual begins to view the situation accurately, he will take steps to change his attitude, his priorities, and his lifestyle. In this type of group setting, the individual is confronted by both staff members and the other patients on the unit. This creates an environment in which the patients and staff "act as a mirror" to make the individual more aware of when he is reverting to drug-related patterns and behaviors.

3. Skill-Oriented Groups

The patient needs to learn how to live sober and deal with people and daily situations without resorting to using alcohol and drugs again. Such groups as Assertive Training, Recovery Planning, Feelings Groups, Men's and Women's Groups, Relaxation and Psychodrama help the individual master more effectively a variety of issues that may prove to be difficult or problematic in early recovery. In addition to didactic presentations, there is much opportunity to practice and role-play these issues. During the later stages of treatment, the patient has signouts outside the hospital milieu. These skill groups prepare the individual to deal with situations in new ways when they return to the community. Conversely, time periods outside the hospital provide some important "behavioral samples" which clarify the individual's specific "vulnerabilities" regarding recovery, and what skills need to be strengthened prior to discharge.

4. Individual Psychotherapy and Counseling

This component aids the program's ability to individualize treatment. These one-to-one sessions with the doctor and addiction counselor allow close monitoring of the individual's status and clinical progress. Special attention can be given to any specific problems concerning anxiety, depression, self-esteem, sexual, interpersonal, family or job. These individual issues need to be carefully entwined in a manner which enhances rather than detracts from the overall thrust of the chemical dependency treatment. Delineation of the individual's psychological or family problems begins a process of self-examination and improved coping that could be continued on an outpatient basis if needed.

5. Family Meetings and Family Education Program

Family participation is an extremely crucial part of the treatment process. Since the patient may be unwilling or unable to disclose certain information about his previous behavior or previous functioning, the family can provide significant background information which provides a broader view of the patient's family's clinical situation. When an individual has a substance abuse problem, the repercussions in the family system are often intense and devastating. Family members become confused, frustrated, and angry because they do not know how to deal with the problem. They often are torn between "writing off" the addict and being overly protective. Tension levels in the family often increase as family members become increasingly polarized as to which approach should be used. The more information the family has concerning the addiction process and how it affects the addict and the family, the easier it is for the family to set limits on the addict in a supportive but firm fashion. In addition, the family helps with discharge planning. They delineate potential problem areas that need to be anticipated following the patient's discharge from the hospital. In addition to the factual information, the families learn about the addiction process, they learn how they themselves can obtain help and support to deal with the ongoing recovery process.

The CDTU has an elaborate Family Night Program every Monday night. There is a brief orientation for family members who are attending the program for the first time. A major portion of the evening is devoted to educating the family about selected topics in addiction. Support is also provided for family members by staff and the other families. Family members are encouraged to participate in family-oriented self-help groups, such as Alanon and Naranon. The patients then join the family group to discuss their progress and additional related issues.

6. Narcotics Anonymous and Alcoholics Anonymous Participation

The self-help fellowships are seen as the basic foundation for the recovery process. The groups provide support, guidance and encouragement to the individual in coping with the problems inherent to the early recovery process. Emotional, family and interpersonal problems which were avoided during active addiction, or handled only within an intoxicated stated, must now be faced without the use of alcohol and drugs. Receiving support and guidance from those who have learned to deal previously with the situations which occur in early sobriety facilitates the individual's ability to effectively respond to this difficult period of adjustment and learning.

The patients attend at least 8 Narcotics Anonymous or Alcoholics Anonymous meetings per week, and as their treatment progresses, they become increasingly involved in Fellowship activities. They talk with members of the recovering community at the meetings, after these meetings, and even on the telephone. They are actively taught how to use the Fellowship — as opposed to merely being a spectator in the process.

In the later phases of treatment, the patient is expected to spend time outside of the hospital with NA or AA contacts. Such participation is seen as quite crucial in aiding the transition from protected hospital environment back to the community.

Role of the Interdisciplinary Team

The doctors, MDs or PhDs, assess the individual's progress and diagnose other psychiatric issues if necessary. They orchestrate the treatment process and coordinate necessary psychological, neurological or medical issue interventions. The nursing staff, in conjunction with the hospital's internist, monitor the medical status and the medical needs of the individual including detoxification at the time of admission.

The drug counselors run many of the group therapies and many of the educational groups. They focus on the "First Step" issues, and relate the patient's loss of control regarding their drug usage and the consequences that the addiction has had on the individual's life and functioning. They also help facilitate the individual's involvement with the Narcotics Anonymous and Alcoholics Anonymous Fellowships.

The social worker serves as the liaison between the family, the patient and the treatment team. She is responsible for planning and implementing the family education program and the individual family sessions. The Head Nurse, the nursing staff and mental health workers lead and co-lead a variety of therapy and educational groups. They are also responsible for the ongoing milieu and the general tone of the treatment environment. Treatment is being given "24 hours a day" and not only when the individual is in formal group sessions.

The hospital's chaplain presents a group on the spiritual aspects of the recovery process. Clearly, this interdisciplinary team meshes many different components of this treatment process into a comprehensive and multifaceted intervention.

Activity Therapy in a Drug Treatment Program

There are many aspects of activity therapy that are relevant to this type of drug treatment program.

a. *Vocational Planning and Counseling.* Given that the addict is often involved in a deviant lifestyle, or has been in an underachieving vocational status, the individual in treatment often is interested in seeking new, more constructive vocational directions. Vocational planning counseling is available if needed, although it is cautioned that the individual should not make too many drastic changes in the early period of recovery. Nonetheless, such information can be useful in the long-term planning of treatment priorities.

b. *Recreational Therapy*. Certainly in this very highly structured confrontative and active milieu it is important to have recreational outlets. This serves to balance the patient's daily schedule and to provide a healthy "escape valve" for the individual and the group. In addition, the patient needs to learn new recovery alternatives to his previous drug-related activities. Recovering addicts often have little understanding of how to use leisure time, given that much of their time was spent in acquiring or using drugs.

Groups related to examining the addict's value system may also be useful. These individuals often see drug-related activities as exciting and fashionable and more societally approved activities as boring and "uncool." Being able to accept a more societally approved activity and enjoy these activities will be helpful to their recovery and to their becoming a more well-balanced individual.

c. *Expressive Art Therapies*. Movement and art therapy can aid the individual in experiencing, labeling, and dealing with feelings that may be difficult to express in a more traditional verbally-oriented treatment modality. Given that years of drug usage and drug-related behaviors tend to make the individual emotionally barren or "dead," becoming more aware of their internal experience can be a most useful adjunct to the recovery process.

d. *Occupational Therapy*. A strong occupational therapy program can strengthen and expand the types of skills taught in a drug treatment program. Activities that help the individual become more aware of his daily living functioning, his self-esteem needs and his means of relating to others can be useful in underscoring the nature of the deficits needing attention in the recovery process.

Such groups and activities can greatly augment the comprehensive intervention detailed previously. A drug treatment program needs to do more than detoxify the individual. Treatment should address how the individual can most effectively reenter society as a sober drug-free functioning individual. Such activities can open up new directions for the person, strengthen coping skills to deal with a variety of interpersonal situations, develop awareness of feelings, and successfully move towards future goals. If the recovering addict does not see a relatively happy, healthy future "on the horizon," it is unlikely that he will put in the work necessary to become drug-free and to make the changes in the lifestyle that are being advocated. Activities therapy is an essential part of dealing with the "whole person" and preparing the recovering addict to deal with the complex situations he will face when he leaves the relatively safe hospital environment.

REFERENCES

Bratter, T.E., Pennacchia, M.C., & Gauya, D.C. (1985). From Methadone to Abstinence. In T.E. Bratter & G.G. Forrest, (eds.). *Alcoholism and Substance Abuse*.

Cohen, S. (1985). *Substance Abuse Problems: New Issues for the 1980's*. New York: Haworth Press.

Dole, V.P. & Nyswander, M. (1976). Methadone maintenance treatment: a ten year perspective. *Journal of the American Medical Association. 235*, 2117-2119.

Forrest, Gary G. (1985). Psychodynamically oriented treatment of alcoholism and substance abuse. In T.E. Bratter & G.G. Forrest (eds.). *Alcoholism and Substance Abuse*. New York: Free Press.

Klein, J.M. & Miller, S.I. (1986). Three approaches to the treatment of drug addiction. *Hospital and Community Psychiatry. 37*:11, 1083-1985.

Milam, J.R. & Ketcham, K. (1983). *Under the Influence*. New York: Bantam Books.

Marlatt, G.A. (1978). Craving for alcohol, loss of control, and relapse: a cognitive behavioral analysis. In P.E. Nathan, G.A. Marlatt, and T. Loberg (eds.). *Alcoholism: New Directors In Behavioral Research and Treatment*. New York: Plenum Press.

Narcotics Anonymous (1984). California: World Services Office.

Ethnographic Interview: An Occupational Therapy Needs Assessment Tool for American Indian and Alaska Native Alcoholics

Barbara K. Lange, MOT

SUMMARY. For an occupational therapist unfamiliar with a culturally diverse treatment population, ethnographic interview is described as an appropriate method for assessing client group needs. This study describes the use of ethnographic interview as a tool which was culturally sensitive to the occupational behaviors of American Indians and Alaska Natives of the Northwest involved in drug and alcohol treatment. Results of the interviews helped the researcher identify sociocultural factors in the acquisition and maintenance of maladaptive behaviors. Recurring themes of the extended family network, the strength and complexity of social norms and codes, and the pervasiveness of alcohol use among this population are described in review of the literature and results of the interviews. Results of the Tennessee Self-Concept Scale revealed an overall

---

Barbara K. Lange is affiliated with the Occupational Therapy Department, University of Utah Hospital, 50 N. Medical Drive, Salt Lake City, UT 84132.

The author would like to thank the following for their encouragement, support, and patience: Juli Evans, George Tomlin, and George Guilmet; David Whitehead; and the staff of the Puyallup Tribal Treatment Center. The author would also like to acknowledge her deepest appreciation and respect for the American Indians and Alaska Natives who so carefully taught her not to ask Why but to instead observe How.

This paper was submitted in partial fulfillment of the requirements for the degree of Master of Occupational Therapy from the University of Puget Sound, Tacoma, WA.

measure of self-esteem significantly lower than that of the normed population, and generally supported rehabilitation issues originally identified by the literature and expanded on in the interviews. Implications for treatment discuss acceptance of the therapist by members of the culture, the concept of noninterference, the role of purposeful activity, cultural identification and assimilation, and the use of group work.

Assessing the needs of diverse cultural groups, such as the American Indians and Alaska Natives of the Northwest, is an important skill for any therapist entering an unfamiliar cultural setting, attempting to define and address the occupational issues of that culture.

Needs assessment will help the therapist respond to the actual needs of the client and not just to treatment needs as perceived by the health care professional (U.S. Dept. Health, Education, and Welfare, 1977). Standards of what is good or healthy may be unconsciously biased by the dominant cultural values of the health care worker (Clark, 1983; Leininger, 1978; Murillo-Rhode, 1979).

For an occupational therapist unfamiliar with a culturally diverse treatment population, ethnographic interview is an appropriate tool for assessing client group needs. Ethnography is the work of defining a culture. Unlike standard research, ethnography does not collect data from people for the purpose of testing an imposed hypothesis. Instead, ethnography seeks to understand the meaning people assign to objects and events in their daily lives. For health professionals, ethnography provides a method for examining health and disease from the patient's point of view, regardless of cultural background.

Since occupational therapy ". . . seeks to promote maximum competence in occupational performance" (Rogers, 1982, p. 34) therapists need to understand the values and traditions of their American Indian and Alaska Native clients to assess accurately their needs and provide culturally appropriate treatment. Anthropological studies have shown that patients may temporarily abandon their own health care practices and beliefs to satisfy health care workers, but will ultimately reject imposed treatment regimes which run counter to internalized cultural values (Leininger, 1978).

PURPOSE OF THE STUDY

The purpose of this study was to implement an occupational therapy needs assessment which was culturally sensitive to the occupational behaviors of Northwest American Indians and Alaska Natives involved in drug and alcohol treatment. This assessment fulfills two purposes: it describes a process which any occupational therapist, newly challenged by an unfamiliar cultural setting, can use to help identify issues of cultural and treatment relevance, and; having been applied to a large group of Indians recently involved in alcohol treatment, offers a broad base of knowledge about a peer group, from which a therapist can identify or compare individual client dysfunction.

REVIEW OF THE LITERATURE

Native Values, Beliefs and Practices

In an attempt to describe a few of the more salient traditional American Indian and Alaska Native values and practices, the author acknowledges the risk of stereotyping. Because of cultural diversity among historically distinct tribal groups, "the value orientations related to productivity, self-maintenance, and leisure are culturally specific to some degree" (Skawski, 1987, p. 38). Concepts of sharing, cooperation, family, noninterference, time, learning style, and spirituality should be considered a characterization of typical group values and corresponding behavior.

"The concept of sharing is deeply ingrained among Native Americans who hold it in greater esteem than the white American ethic of saving" (Lewis & Ho, 1975, p. 379). Indians derive little status from the permanent accumulation of material goods. Historically in the Northwest culture area the Indian potlatch, a festive gathering of friends and neighbors in which an individual would distribute his accumulation of food, blankets or other useful items, is an example of the importance of sharing (Jilek-Aall, 1981).

Cooperation, patience, and nonaggression are important values among Native Americans. Unlike members of the white majority, Indians and Eskimos do not publicly emphasize individual achievements, and often do not feel as comfortable when encouraged to compete with peers (Weiringa & McColl, 1987). Skills tend to be used to contribute to the well-being of the family and tribe, and not for personal gain.

"To be really poor in the Indian world is to be without relatives" (Primeaux, 1977, p. 92). The extended family and the tribe are of foremost importance to the traditional Indian. Children are highly valued, loved and wanted. Elders are respected for their wisdom and expertise in traditional matters, and are valued for their ability to pass down their knowledge through myth, legend and folklore (Primeaux, 1977; Weiringa & McColl, 1987). Within the family, independence is encouraged. Children often eat, sleep, and play without seeking permission of their parents. They are usually free to explore their surroundings and are rarely told they cannot do something. Young children are protected from danger by having the danger removed. Older children are told about possible consequences of an act or decision, but are then "left free to make their choice" (Backrup, 1979, p. 22).

Freedom to explore the environment is also an essential component of Indian learning style. Guilmet's review of the literature describing American Indian learning styles contrasts the way Indian children learn at home or within their native cultural environment, with teaching strategies typically used in white school systems (1985). Historical and contemporary evidence indicates that when learning technical knowledge or skills Indian children may receive verbal guidance from elders or teachers only after a lengthy period of observation of the task. Indian children may then experiment with trial and error to master the task independently, before presenting their skill or product for approval. For non-Indian children the long period of observation may be replaced by elaborate verbal instructions which describe the task in detail. Indian children, for whom sharp observational skills are culturally prominent, are at a specific disadvantage in white school systems where language is the primary teaching/learning modality. Also at odds with the white classroom emphasis on competition, verbalization, and individual achievement, are the Indian values of cooperation, nonaggression, and patience.

Patience is taught early to Indian children. They may play in the midst of a group of adults, but know not to interrupt their conversation. Indian adults may not respond to tantrums or outbursts by children, who are taught at a young age to control their emotions. Indian children are treated with the same respect and consideration they are taught to show others (Good Tracks, 1973). Child-rearing practices of Native Americans are largely based on the important concept of noninterference.

In American Indian society attempts to persuade or counsel another person, even to keep that person from doing something dangerous or foolish, are considered rude and will not be tolerated. White health care workers, teachers, and social workers are taught to "help" others through advising and counseling. These actions may be interpreted by Indians as "meddling," and they will usually not respond to such interference (Lewis & Ho, 1975).

Traditional Indians also differ from white Americans in their concept of time. Time, as structured by a twenty-four hour clock, traditionally had no objective value to Indians. Their concept of time was a cyclical one based on naturally recurring phenomena; sunrise, sunset, days, nights, moons (months), and seasons (Lewis, 1975). A difference in time orientation also applies to orientation to the future. Whereas the white middle class is preoccupied with "saving for the future" and the "future of their children," many Indians are oriented to the present. In their earlier subsistence lifestyle, work was done to satisfy a present need, rather than long term future security (Jilek-Aall, 1981). The mother earth provided all that was needed, and maintaining balance with nature by using only what was needed and saving for the next winter was in itself enough of a consideration for the future (Baker, 1982).

"American Indians have a profound spiritual relationship with nature and mother earth" (Backrup, 1979, p. 22). Maintaining harmony with spiritual forces which underlie and pervade nature and the perceived world is seen as the basis of health. "To the American Indian, 'medicine' means more than just the treatment of diseases and healing of injuries. There is little distinction between medicine and religion; they are aspects of the same thing" (Primeaux, 1977, p. 91). A primary purpose of Indian religions is to support a balance between the individual, other people, nature, and the spirit world. Traditionally, illness was treated in part by a shaman whose behaviors encompassed those of the contemporary physician, psychiatrist, and spiritual leader. The shaman, or medicine man possesses supernatural powers obtained through contacts with the "underworld" or communication with a guiding spirit (Jilek, 1982). Although shamanistic healing rituals vary from tribe to tribe, medicine men and medicine women consider the health of the individual to include his/her mind, body, and a personal relationship with the environment. They do not dichotomize the world into mental versus physical illness. The treatment process, which could include the ritualistic use of herbs, as well as ceremonial dancing or praying, is geared toward restoring the person's harmony and oneness with the natural and spiritual world. Tribal religions provided a code for acceptable behavior, social organization "which contributed to an understanding of the meaning of life" (Mitchell & Patch, 1986, p. 129), and the means (ceremonies, rituals, and treatments) for preventing and dealing with individual or social dysfunction.

It must be understood that what has just been presented is a very general, brief description of a few traditional American Indian and Alaska Native beliefs and values. Although many tribal values and traditions are intact (to various degrees) and are expressed through individual and group behaviors, the problems of contemporary American Indians and Alaska Natives closely reflect the plight of the urban poor in America.

On many reservations, boredom, the absence of traditional roles, and the lack of opportunity to obtain white society's well-advertised "good life," exacerbate and perpetuate alcohol abuse, dissolution of the family, and general hopelessness among Indians. Rural Indians who do obtain an education or career opportunity off the reservation may experience conflict in trying to balance their two roles (Jilek-Aall, 1981).

American Indians living on urban reservations experience high unemployment, inadequate housing, and high rates of alcohol and drug abuse. Child neglect, spouse abuse, and high divorce rates indicate a general breakdown of the family unit (Guilmet, 1984). Urban Indians who have moved off their rural reservations are often deprived of supportive extended family networks. They may feel equally alienated from both their native culture and the white majority culture. Walker (1981) points out that in view of the steadily increasing migration of Indians into cities such as Los Angeles,

Chicago, Minneapolis and Seattle, urban Indian alcohol programs must be designed to help Indians synthesize the values of the two cultures in which they live.

It is important for the occupational therapist to acknowledge the cultural traditions of American Indian and Alaska Native clients. The history and traditions of the aboriginal Indian are the basis for many of the occupational behaviors of contemporary urban and reservation-based American Indians. Because the health needs of each ethnic minority are unique, the therapist who has knowledge of various cultural groups is in a better position to communicate effectively with and treat his or her minority clients.

Scope of the Problem

To say that alcohol abuse is the number one health problem of American Indians and Alaska Natives (Baker, 1982; Beauvais & LaBoueff, 1985; Levy & Kunitz, 1974; Weibel-Orlando, 1984) understates the extent of the problem. The effects of alcohol abuse are far-reaching and perpetuate a cycle of family dissolution, economic depression, and community anomie. Indian people die younger than any other ethnic group in the country, with five of the ten leading causes of death directly related to alcohol. Alcohol is involved in 75% of all fatal accidents, 80% of all suicides, and 90% of all homicides (Kauffman, 1986). Mail (1985) reported that alcohol abuse is a main factor in the removal of Indian children from their homes, marital problems, spouse and child neglect, increased rates of infant morbidity caused by fetal alcohol syndrome, employment instability, and "complications in one's spiritual life" (p. 3). In their survey of Indian youth attending rural reservation schools, Oetting, Beauvais and Goldstein (1981) found that drug and alcohol use is well-established among children in the 4th-7th grades.

The almost overwhelming scope of the Indian alcohol problem is compounded by notoriously ineffective alcohol treatment programs designed for and by white people (Kivlahan, Walker, Donovan, & Mischke, 1985; Query, 1985; Weibel-Orlando, 1984; Weibel-Orlando, Weisner, & Long, 1984). In response to a specific need, cultural identification and prevention strategies are currently being emphasized by many federally funded, tribally operated Indian alcohol treatment programs (Albaugh & Anderson, 1974; Hall, 1986; "Self Help," 1974).

Ceremonial use of the sweat lodge is a cleansing and healing ritual once used by most aboriginal North American tribes. Although use of the sweat lodge had lapsed in many parts of the country, Hall (1986) found it to be an alcohol treatment modality popular among tribal treatment programs. This was particularly true of multitribal programs that also provided client access to the Native American Church, or employed a medicine man on a regular basis. Hall suggested that renewed popularity of the sweat lodge is part of a nativist reform movement which emphasizes Indian self-sufficiency, a return to the spiritual concepts of the pre-European past, and abstinence from alcohol.

Jilek-Aall (1981, p. 156) notes that, "as does the Coast Salish spirit-dancer, the Indian A.A. member counts his age from the day he was 'reborn' into the new way of life." The traditional Indian symbolism being incorporated into A.A. meetings, along with the revival of spirit-dancing, both described by Jilek-Aall, lend further support to the ideology of the pan-Indian movement. Unfortunately, culturally relevant Indian alcohol treatment programs are few in number.

In response to the need for a culturally relevant curriculum, the United Tribes of All Nations Foundation in Seattle, Washington, developed a unique puppetry presentation for children ages five to eleven (1987). The goal of the No! No! Know Puppetry Presentation is to reduce drug and alcohol related problems among the American Indian population by increasing resistance to addiction. Puppets are used to teach children coping skills, self-expression, listening skills, decision making, personal responsibility, and facts about alcohol and drugs. Puppet costumes and characters represent Indian symbols from several tribes, and are used to create and pass on legends and teachings once taught by Indian families.

RESEARCH SETTING

In response to the needs of the 140 tribes it serves, the Puyallup Tribal Treatment Center (PTTC) in Tacoma, Washington, has successfully integrated Western and traditional treatments through the Medicine Wheel approach. This holistic health care approach addresses the social, psychological, physical, and spiritual aspects of a client's illness (Guilmet, 1984). The program, selected in February, 1983 as a model alcoholism program in the Portland Area Indian Health Service Region, offers inpatient, outpatient, follow-up and prevention programs. The center maintains a sweat lodge which is primarily used by inpatient clients. Individual and group counseling, and classes in alcohol and drug education, poetry, and nutrition, emphasize cultural awareness and exploration. The variety of services and strategies used by the treatment center allows staff to effectively treat rural and urban Indians from ethnographically diverse tribal cultures.

To ensure comprehensive treatment programming, and to fulfill contract requirements with the three state and federal agencies providing monies, the Puyallup Tribal Treatment Center would like to incorporate occupational therapy services into its treatment program. An occupational behaviors needs assessment helped the therapist identify sociocultural factors in the acquisition and maintenance of problem behaviors. Methods may now be developed which facilitate "unlearning" of maladaptive behaviors and the "learning" of new or adaptive behaviors.

METHODOLOGY

Ethnography may be used to expand the traditional psychosocial needs assessment format. The therapist/ethnographer spent casual time in the rehabilitation setting building a rapport with clients based on trust, cooperation, and mutual exploration. This researcher reviewed relevant literature, but also volunteered many hours at PTTC, the site of the research project. Hours spent playing volleyball, tutoring GED students, and just "hanging out" allowed the researcher to establish a greater rapport and provided more information than would have been possible had the researcher chosen to maintain her professional role as therapist. Establishing informal lines of communication is the initial step in ethnographic interview research, and is recommended by Westermeyer (1976) as appropriate to the development of strategies for cross-cultural treatment of chemical dependency.

To begin the actual interview process, five American Indians of different ages and backgrounds were individually asked to, "tell a little bit about yourself" or, "describe how you ended up here." These broad, general, "Grand Tour" questions encouraged PTTC clients to give a verbal description of significant features in their cultural scene (Spradley, 1979). During these initial interviews it was important for the therapist/researcher to make a verbatim record of what clients were saying. Although not every word was transcribed, noted phrases were reported using the client's own terms. The researcher was tempted to summarize or unconsciously translate native terms into seemingly more meaningful professional jargon, but this would have been a mistake. Words are the tools and symbols of a culture, and as such hold value as a key to that culture. One young Yakima man repeatedly referred to those in his family who still "practiced." Further conversation and presentation of the term in context revealed a social code behind the meaning of "practice" that a simple meaning translation of "drink alcohol" would not have yielded. Once broad areas of cultural and personal significance were described by the informants, the therapist/researcher used subsequent interviews to ask more specific questions concerning particular events, places, or situations.

Asking for examples, descriptions of specific experiences, and for projection into hypothetical situations are typical ways ethnographers grade for more specific information (Spradley, 1979). This researcher used second and third interviews to ask for more information about family issues, jobs, or events initially mentioned by the informants. During these continuing interviews the researcher avoided asking "why" questions. Questions that ask why ("why did the court take your children away from you?," "why do you drink?") contain a judgemental component (Spradley, 1979). They indicate to the informant that they have not been clear, have not provided the right answer, or that their actions were not understood or condoned by the interviewer.

Common events or issues raised by the five initial informants are defined by ethnographers as cultural meaning systems. On review, the researcher was able to define relationships between common events and issues identified by informants. From groups of "answers" provided by the five initial informants, the researcher designed eleven specific questions to be used in a larger scale, more traditional interview series (see Appendix A). For the purpose of gathering information for use in that particular treatment setting, the above outlined process alone would have been effective as a needs assessment process. Further interviewing of a larger peer group was necessary only for the comparison of the results of ethnographic interview with review of the literature and results of the Tennessee Self-Concept Scale.

The final stage in the research process was the interview set of thirty-one American Indians and Alaska Natives (21 men and 10 women) undergoing alcohol and drug rehabilitation at the Puyallup Tribal Treatment Center, in Tacoma, Washington. All clients participating in the study were federally recognized as American Indian or Alaska Native, and represented nineteen different Northwest and Midwest tribes. Informant ages ranged from 21 to 51 years, with a median age of 31.8 years. Each interview began with administration of the Tennessee Self-Concept Scale. This scale, which measures several components of self-esteem, has high test-retest reliability and has been normed on Indian populations. The eleven interview questions reflected intra- and interpersonal issues regarding personal goals, family relations, and strategies for meeting needs.

RESULTS AND DISCUSSION

In response to the interview question, "As far as drinking goes, will your family help you stay sober, or will they hinder you?," 80% of all respondents said that their families would help them maintain sobriety. Of this subgroup, 32% said that while their families would be generally supportive, many family members, by virtue of their own drinking habits, would also hinder efforts to stay sober. While only one respondent described family as a purely negative influence on sobriety, 16% of respondents described incidents in which family members tried to discourage them from undergoing alcohol or drug treatment. To her father and brother's allegation that, "You drink, sure, but you're not treatment material," one young Sioux woman responded, "This is for me to do. . . . Please don't try to talk me out of it." Later she commented, "I have learned that my brother has a drinking problem also. . . . The problem was getting a little too close to him by his sister coming to treatment." A Yakima man described his road trip to Tacoma, accompanied by his father and his father's friend, this way: "They tried to talk me out of it. They said, 'You don't need treatment. You can handle it.' Then on the way we started drinking, and kept drinking for seven or eight days. Finally I couldn't stand it anymore and went to detox, and then treatment.''

Other examples of the importance of family surfaced throughout the various interview questions. When specifically asked what would help them stay sober after leaving the treatment center, 19% of the interviewed population answered: increases in family communication and interaction, the emotional support of the family, and repair of family ties damaged by alcoholism. Increased familial affiliation was one of four major items identified as necessary to achieving and maintaining permanent sobriety.

Forty-five percent of informants said they needed the support of other alcoholics to help them stay sober. They specifically described a determination to use Alcoholics Anonymous (A.A.) and A.A. sponsors as personal resources. Many informants considered A.A. meetings a way to meet people who did not drink, and a way to structure time formerly spent drinking.

Thirty-five percent of the interviewed population defined steady work as helpful to maintaining sobriety. Many respondents said that seasonal employment, lack of opportunity on the reservation, or inadequate training in competitive urban job markets, decreased their sense of self-worth and ability to meet basic financial needs. Few interviewed described a desire for middle-class material comforts, or occupational status. Most spoke of work as a way to meet basic financial needs and achieve a sense of productivity. Some of these people viewed work as a means to another end. They saw the skills developed and the money earned from working as something they could bring back to their people as a contribution to the common good. One woman wanted to pursue a nursing career and bring her skills back to her reservation in South Dakota. Another man was applying for a vocational course in small business management. He wanted to use those skills on his reservation where several federally funded economic growth projects had failed due to tribal inability to manage project operations. And yet another person wished to use his earnings to sponsor a home youth basketball team. Work is valued by American Indian and Alaska Native populations, but for reasons less centered around personal identity or gain, than in the majority culture.

Other small percentages of informants said that the drug Antabuse, increased assertiveness and self-expression, prayer, and/or a sober spouse would help them maintain permanent sobriety. Many Indians (19%) identified a stable environment, away from their old crowd, as a prerequisite for sobriety. "It scares me that I'm going back to an environment that's not stable — my reservation," said a Colville youth. And a Spokane said, "That's one of the big things, all my friends (on the reservation) drink."

When asked how not drinking will specifically affect their social lives, 58% of informants said that their social life would be drastically changed and would be based on forming new friendships with nondrinkers, and/or setting limits with old friends. A few in this group (27%) said they really did not have a social life, that alcohol had consumed them and their relationships. Or as one man said, "When I was younger they used to have that song, 'All My Rowdy Friends Are Settled Down.' Most of my rowdy friends are dead . . . due to alcoholism."

Twenty-five percent of all interviewed said their social lives would not change at all. Many in this group said they could go back to the same setting and not be pressured to drink, and one man described his sobriety as a potential source of status among members of his tribe. The differences here seemed to depend on the specific situation or reservation to which the client was returning.

Many of the American Indian and Alaska Native clients interviewed (29%) looked forward to participating in activities they had abandoned during their drinking careers. These activities included hunting, fishing, war dancing, sports, artistic endeavors, church activities, and of course, increased time with children and family.

Analysis of the Tennessee Self-Concept Scale (TSCS) revealed an overall measure of self-esteem (Total Positive Score) among PTTC clients significantly lower than that of the normed population. T-tests of the eight subsections comprising the Total Positive Score identified scores significantly lower in every area (see Table 1).

The group mean for the Total Variability score was 50.226, compared to a normed mean of 48.53 [$t(df\ 30) = 5.68$, $p < .5773$].

TABLE 1

COMPARISON OF THE RESULTS OF THE TENNESSEE
SELF-CONCEPT SCALE: SAMPLE TO POPULATION

SUBTESTS	SAMPLE MEAN	STANDARD DEVIATION	NORMED MEAN	P <
Self-satisfaction	92.226	12.476	103.67	0.001
Behavior	102.710	13.967	115.01	0.001
Identity	111.581	16.035	127.1	0.001
Physical self	61.645	8.468	71.78	0.001
Moral-ethical	61.065	7.655	70.33	0.001
Personal self	57.774	7.205	64.55	0.001
Family	61.097	11.435	70.83	0.001
Social self	61.516	7.393	68.14	0.001
*Total Positive	306.258	33.402	345.57	0.001
Total V	50.226	16.627	48.53	0.5773
Self-criticism	34.323	5.275	35.54	0.2063

This score suggests that the tested population was fairly well integrated in that they did not separate their actions from themselves. The Indian and Alaska Native population seem to lack a sense of personal definition, and harbor negative images of themselves and their behaviors (as described by low subtest scores in Identity, Behavior, and Self-Satisfaction). Results of the variability score may also mean that they are consistent in accepting their alcoholism as an internal condition, not something removed or external to their being. An internalized dissatisfaction with self and behavior may be a step toward acceptance of responsibility for self and behavior, an important factor in the self-healing processes in alcohol and drug rehabilitation.

In general, results of the Tennessee Self-Concept Scale reconfirmed rehabilitation issues, including social and personal conflicts, identified in ethnographic interviews. American Indian and Alaska Native values, alluded to in review of the literature, laid the historical foundation for issues essentially brought to life through ethnographic interview.

For example, analysis of the TSCS provided significantly low Family subtest scores. This generally reflects group feelings of inadequacy or deflated worth as family members. It suggests that familial cohesion or sense of affiliation, described by the literature as important cultural foundations, may be insecure within this group. But nowhere is the complexity of relationships in the extended American Indian and Alaska Native family described as thoroughly as in the ethnographic interview responses to related questions. Informant responses suggest a complex relationship between societal norms and personal goal issues that quantitative research methods may have failed to elicit. "I don't see Indian actors, or doctors, or athletes. . . . You'll never see an Indian president. Indians on the reservations I've been on, they don't care what goes on in this world. They just accept their surroundings and where they live. They're just Indians."

Recurring themes of the expanded family network, the strength and complexity of social norms and codes, and the pervasiveness of alcohol use among the native population combine with native learning style and occupational therapy theory base to suggest implications for treatment.

IMPLICATIONS FOR TREATMENT

Occupational therapists have a broad knowledge and skill base with which they can offer meaningful therapy to American Indian and Alaska Native alcoholics. Based on information from the literature and the ethnographic interview, the following suggestions are offered.

Before an incoming therapist can hope to be an effective provider of meaningful therapy, she or he must gain the acceptance and respect of his or her client population. In an Indian community where time may be atypically structured, and the daily pace may be unregulated by work commitments, a therapist who sets out to structure time, organize the environment, and objectify activities and behaviors, may be perceived with suspicion or mistrust by an American Indian or Alaska Native population. The therapist must take the time to become familiar and comfortable with the existing native social framework, before he or she will be accepted and turned to as a resource. The therapist must not be tempted to challenge or aggressively change the existing social structure. The therapist who emphasizes his or her professional role and educational status may be ignored by American Indian and Alaska Native clients who hold little regard for such credentials. A therapist is more likely to earn respect for his or her show of patience, willingness to share, and nonjudgemental or noncoercive attitudes. Acceptance is a slow process, and a therapist's intrinsic patience will be tested.

Group work is a natural medium for occupational therapists and this particular client population. The therapist can build on American Indian and Alaska Native values of cooperation and sharing. Group work allows members to increase self-esteem by contributing to a common goal or outcome. In harmony with native learning styles, group tasks allow individual members to observe new skills without feeling threatened or pushed to perform, or compete against peers. The therapist, by assuming an equal role of participant-observer, can model for group members, and should allow, but not push, other members to assume leadership roles. In group work, as in any aspect of therapy with American Indian and Alaska Native clients, the therapist may need to repress his or her desire to control, or instigate client participation. Respecting the principle of noninterference, the therapist should provide the opportunity for skill development or exploration, but may wish to refrain from prematurely promoting client action. Those who wish to participate may, when they are ready. Those who choose not to participate should not be chastised for their behavior. Therapists may need to abandon preconceived notions of what is productive, assertive, or healthy behavior, and learn to respect unique cultural norms. For example, among American Indians, direct eye-contact may be considered a rude or intimidating behavior. They may show respect by not staring or looking directly at others (Lewis, 1975).

Successful group work requires that the therapist be subtle in his or her intervention, and rely on indirect means of group influence. Therapists with a repertoire of psychoanalytical exercises designed to facilitate human growth and personal development through sharing and analysis of personal experience, may be rebuffed by the native population. American Indians and Alaska Natives may be uncomfortable discussing issues and events usually kept within the family. A therapist who pushes for personal disclosure, particularly in a group setting, does not understand the native concept of noninterference.

Much of occupational therapy theory base emphasizes the promotion and maintenance of health through purposeful activity. The therapist working with American Indian clients may be surprised to discover that this premise is not universal, and may be in fact a product of the professional culture. Weiringa and McColl (1987) point out that time spent with others in silence, normal in Native culture, may be interpreted by Western standards as inactivity. Therapists must accept the contemplative and patient nature of the Indian culture, and be aware of American Indian and Alaska Native tendencies to accept and endure the painful aspects of life as well as the good. Native spiritual beliefs, and a strong sense of social and environmental interdependence, encourage patience in problem resolution, and may contradict Western tendencies to change a situation by assertive action.

Occupational therapists working with American Indians and Alaska Natives in an alcohol treatment center, or any setting, should recognize and try to work within the influence of the extended family network and peer social code. Habilitation and rehabilitation must be offered in a context relevant to the individual, and should include family participation when possible. The occupational therapist should encourage client cultural identification as a way to increase self-esteem and sense of affiliation, necessary components of health. At the same time, the therapist should not assume that his or her American Indian or Alaska Native clients will overtly express any of the values identified here. Many American Indians have grossly assimilated the white culture and some may have no individual need to explore their historical past or subcultural present. By not making assumptions about a culture, the therapist can encourage members of the culture to identify relevant issues, questions, and answers. To facilitate this, the therapist should treat his or her American Indian and Alaska Native client as an equal, and provide a nonjudgemental, loosely structured environment for therapy.

In this study, the ethnographic interview provided an in-depth contemporary perspective on American Indian and Alaska Native culture that a literature review could only lay a foundation for and a standardized testing tool could only scratch the surface of.

Alaska Natives and American Indians have much to teach health professionals. By assimilating American Indian and Alaska Native values of patience, interdependence, and observational learning style, occupational therapists can expand their understanding of holism and be effective mentors of American Indian and Alaska Native wellness.

REFERENCES

Albaugh, B., & Anderson, P. (1974). Peyote in the treatment of alcoholism among American Indians. *American Journal of Psychiatry. 131*, 1247-1251.

Backrup, R. (1979). Implementing quality health care for the American Indian patient. *Washington State Journal of Nursing-Special Supplement.* 20-24.

Baker, J. (1982). Alcoholism and the American Indian. *Alcoholism, Development, Consequences and Interventions* (pp. 239-248). C.V. Mosby Co.

Beauvais, F., & LaBoueff, S. (1985). Drug and alcohol abuse intervention in American Indian communities. *International Journal of the Addictions. 20*, 139-171.

Clark, M. (1983). Cultural context of medical practice. *Western Journal of Medicine. 139*, 239-248.

Good Tracks, J. (1973). Native American non-interference. *Social Work. 18*, 30-34.

Guilmet, G. (1984). Health care and health care seeking strategies among Puyallup Indians. *Culture, Medicine and Psychiatry. 8*, 349-369.

Guilmet, G. (1985). The nonverbal American Indian child in the classroom: A survey. ERIC Clearinghouse on Rural Education and Small Schools: New Mexico State University.

Hall, R. (1986). Distribution of the sweat lodge in alcohol treatment programs. Comparative perspectives from Europe and America. *Annals of the New York Academy of Sciences. 472*, 169-177.

Jilek, W. (1982). *Indian Healing-Shamanistic Ceremonialism in the Pacific Northwest Today*. Hancock House Publishers Ltd.

Jilek-Aall, L. (1981). Acculturation, alcoholism and Indian-style Alcoholics Anonymous. *Journal of Studies on Alcohol. Supplement No. 9*, 143-158.

Kauffman, J. (1986). Indian alcoholism a nat'l plague. *NIHB Health Reporter. 4*, 5-8.

Kivlahan, D., Walker, R., Donovan, D., & Mischke, H. (1985). Detoxification recidivism among urban American Indian alcoholics. *American Journal of Psychiatry. 142*, 1467-1470.

Leininger, M. (1978). Ethnoscience: A promising research approach to improve nursing practice. *Transcultural Nursing: Concepts, Theories, and Practices* (pp. 75-83). John Wiley & Sons.

Levy, J., & Kunitz, S. (1974). *Indian Drinking—Navajo Practices and Anglo-American Theories*. John Wiley & Sons.

Lewis, R., & Ho, M. (1975). Social work with Native Americans. *Social Work.* *20*, 379-382.

Mail, P. (1985). Closing the circle: A prevention model for Indian communities with alcohol problems. *IHS Primary Care Provider. 1*, 2-5.

Mitchell, W., & Patch, K. (1986). Religion, spiritualism, and the recovery of Native American alcoholics. *IHS Primary Care Provider. 11*, 129.

Murillo-Rhode, I. (1979). Cultural sensitivity in the care of the Hispanic patient. *Washington State Journal of Nursing – Special Supplement*, 25-32.

Oetting, E., Beauvais, F., & Goldstein, S. (1982). *Drug Use Among Native American Youth: Summary of Findings (1975-1981).* Western Behavioral Studies, Colorado State University.

Primeaux, M. (1977). Caring for the American Indian patient. *American Journal of Nursing. 77*, 91-94.

Query, J. (1985). Comparative admission and follow-up study of American Indians and whites in a youth chemical dependency unit on the north central plains. *International Journal of the Addictions. 20*, 489-502.

Rogers, J.C. (1982). Order and disorder in medicine and occupational therapy. *American Journal of Occupational Therapy. 36*, 34.

Self-help programs for Indians and Native Alaskans. (1974). *Alcohol and Research World.* Summer, 11-16.

Skawski, K. (1987). Ethnic/racial considerations in occupational therapy. *Occupational Therapy in Health Care. 4*, 37-48.

Spradley, J. (1979). *The Ethnographic Interview.* Holt, Rinehart, and Winston.

United Tribes of all Nations Foundation. (1987, February). No! No! Know puppetry presentation. Youth Education and Prevention. *Symposium conducted by the Northwest Indian Alcohol Coalition*, Blake Island, WA.

U.S. Dept. of Health, Education, and Welfare. (1977). *Needs Assessment Approaches: Concepts and Methods.* Public Health Service.

Walker, R.D. (1981). Treatment strategies in an urban Indian alcoholism program. *Journal of Studies of Alcohol. Supplement No. 9*, 171-184.

Walker, R.D., & Kirvlahan, D. (1984). Definitions, models, and methods in research in sociocultural factors in American Indian alcohol use. *Substance and Alcohol Actions Misuse. 5*, 9-18.

Weibel-Orlando, J.C. (1984). Indian alcoholism treatment programs as flawed rites of passage. *Medical Anthropology Newsletter. 15*, 62-67.

Weibel-Orlando, J.C., Weisner, T., & Long, J. (1984). Urban and rural drinking patterns: Implications for intervention policy development. *Substance and Alcohol Actions/Misuse. 5*, 45-56.

Weiringa, N., & McColl, M. (1987). Implications of the model of human occupation for intervention with Native Canadians. *Occupational Therapy in Health Care. 4*, 73-91.

Westermeyer, J. (1976). Clinical guidelines for the cross-cultural treatment of chemical dependency. *American Journal of Drug and Alcohol Abuse. 3*, 315-322.

APPENDIX A

The Formal Interview Questions

1. What is your definition of an alcoholic?
2. Are you an alcoholic, or do you have a drinking problem?
3. How does drinking make you feel?
4. Now that you have been sober awhile, how do you feel?
5. When you leave here (the treatment center), what would help you stay sober? What skills or support do you need?
6. What do you think is the best way to get that (what client identified in above question)?
7. As far as drinking goes, will your family help you stay sober or will they hinder you?
8. How will not drinking affect your social life?
9. How does your "Indianness" conflict with the non-Indian world? In other words, has being Indian (or Alaska Native) caused any problems for you?
10. Is there anything in this life you would really like to do?
11. What is stopping you from doing that?